Y0-BCU-088

Basic CPT/HCPCS
Coding Exercises
First Edition

Gail I. Smith, MA, RHIA, CCS-P

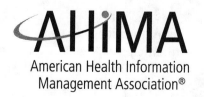

American Health Information
Management Association®

CPT five-digit codes, nomenclature, and other data are the property of the American Medical Association. Copyright ©2008 by the American Medical Association. All rights reserved. No fee schedules, basic unit, relative values, or related listings are included in CPT. *The AMA assumes no liability for the data contained herein.*

This workbook must be used with the current edition of *Current Procedural Terminology* (code changes effective January 1, 2008), published by the American Medical Association (AMA). Any five-digit numeric CPT codes, service descriptions, instructions, and/or guidelines are copyright 2008 (or such other date of publication of CPT as defined in the federal copyright laws) by the AMA.

CPT is a listing of descriptive terms and five-digit numeric identifying codes and modifiers for reporting medical services performed by physicians. This presentation includes only CPT descriptive terms, numeric identifying codes, and modifiers for reporting medical services and procedures that were selected by the American Health Information Management Association (AHIMA) for inclusion in this publication.

AHIMA has selected certain CPT codes and service/procedure descriptions and assigned them to various specialty groups. The listing of a CPT service/procedure description and its code number in this publication does not restrict its use to a particular specialty group. Any procedure/service in this publication may be used to designate the services rendered by any qualified physician.

Copyright ©2008 by the American Health Information Management Association. All rights reserved. No part of this publication may be reproduced, stored in a retrieval system, or transmitted, in any form or by any means, electronic, photocopying, recording, or otherwise, without the prior written permission of the publisher.

The Web sites listed in this book were current and valid as of the date of publication. However, Web page addresses and the information on them may change or disappear at any time and for any number of reasons. The user is encouraged to perform his or her own general Web searches to locate any site addresses listed here that are no longer valid.

ISBN: 1-58426-204-4
ISBN-13: 978-1-58426-204-6

AHIMA Product Number AC210608

Kimberly L. Hines, Project Editor
Katie Greenock, Assistant Editor
Melissa Ulbricht, Editorial/Production Coordinator
Ken Zielske, Director of Publications
Karen M. Kostick, RHIT, CCS, CCS-P, Technical Reviewer
Melanie Endicott, MBA/HCM, RHIA, CCS, CCS-P, Technical Reviewer

American Health Information Management Association
233 North Michigan Avenue, 21st Floor
Chicago, Illinois 60601-5800
www.ahima.org

Contents

About the Author

Gail I. Smith, MA, RHIA, CCS-P, is an associate professor and director of the health information management program at the University of Cincinnati in Cincinnati, Ohio. She has been an HIM professional and educator for more than thirty years. Prior to joining the faculty at the University of Cincinnati, she was director of a health information technology associate degree program and was health information manager in a multihospital healthcare system.

Ms. Smith also is a coding consultant and a frequent presenter at conferences throughout the United States. An active member of the American Health Information Management Association (AHIMA), she has served on the board of directors and several of AHIMA's committees and task forces.

Ms. Smith received a bachelor of science degree in health information management from The Ohio State University in Columbus and a master of arts degree in education from The College of Mt. St. Joseph in Cincinnati.

Preface

This workbook serves as a companion to *Basic CPT/HCPCS Coding* published by the American Health Information Management Association (AHIMA). It is designed to provide additional practice exercises for applying CPT coding guidelines to case studies. In addition, medical terminology is reinforced with matching quizzes and crossword puzzles.

Organization of the Workbook

The workbook follows the same chapter titles as *Basic CPT/HCPCS Coding*. Students are asked to identify the key terms for locating the coding selection (code or range of codes to verify) and subsequent assignment of CPT codes to describe the procedures and services. Actual case studies and operative reports provide an opportunity for students to analyze documentation to support accurate coding selection. In addition, the detailed answer key contains documentation highlighted for better understanding of the relationship between documentation and correct assignment of CPT code(s). The following is a summary of chapter highlights:

Chapter	Title	Activities
1	Introduction to Clinical Coding	Crossword Puzzle Case Studies
2	Application of CPT System	Matching Exercise Referencing *CPT Assistant* Application of CPT Exercises
3	Modifiers	Matching Select Modifier Exercises Coding/Modifier Application Exercises
4	Surgery	Matching Exercises Crossword Puzzles Operative Notes Emergency Department Records Operative Reports Physician Office Records
5	Radiology	Medical Terminology Review Case Studies
6	Pathology & Laboratory	Case Studies
7	Evaluation and Management Services	Case Studies
8	Medicine	Case Studies
9	Anesthesia	Case Studies
10	HCPCS	Case Studies
	Answer Key	Answer Key

Chapter 1

Introduction to Clinical Coding

Chapter 1 provides an overview of coding and its use in the claims submission process. It is vital that the CPT codes and ICD-9-CM codes provided are supported by the documentation in the patient's medical record. The ICD-9-CM diagnosis code should identify why the patient was seeking services (treatment, therapy, etc.), and CPT codes should identify the services that were performed.

In the following case studies, refer to the listed CPT code description, and identify any discrepancies between the CPT code selection and supportive documentation.

Case Study #1

The patient is seen as an outpatient for a bilateral mammogram.

CPT Code: 77055–50

_____

_____

Case Study #2

A physician performs a closed manipulation of a medial malleolus fracture—left ankle.

CPT Code: 27766–LT

_____

_____

Case Study #3

A surgeon performs a cystourethroscopy with dilation of a urethral stricture.

CPT Code: 52341

_____

_____

Case Study #4

The operative report states that the physician performed Strabismus surgery, requiring resection of the medial rectus muscle.

CPT Code: 67314

_____

_____

Case Study #5

A chiropractor documents that he performed osteopathic manipulation on the neck and back (lumbar/thoracic).

CPT Code: 9892

_____

_____

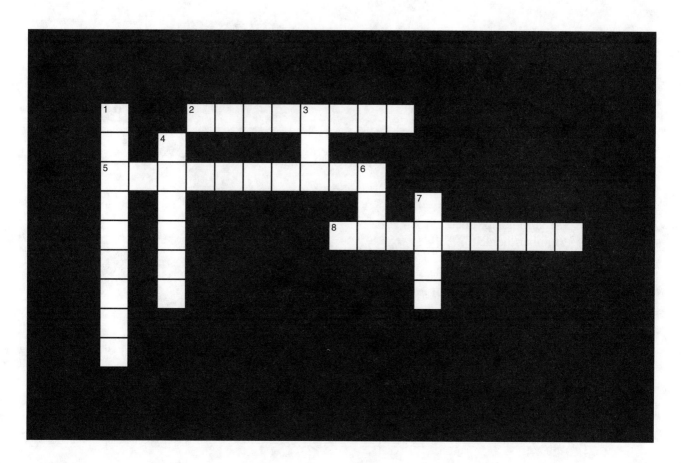

Across

2. Federal insurance for those over age 65
5. Modifier P4 found in this CPT section
8. CT Scans found in this section of CPT

Down

1. Supports medical necessity
3. Agency administers Medicare
4. A new edition of CPT is published _____
6. Organization that publishes CPT
7. Number of digits in CPT code

Chapter 2

Application of the CPT System

Matching Exercise

Match the correct definitions or descriptions.

1. ____ Complete list of modifiers

2. ____ Complete list of add-on codes

3. ____ 82525 Copper

4. ____ Complete list of recent additions, deletions and revisions

5. ____ 1039F Intermittent asthma

A. Appendix B

B. Category II code

C. Appendix D

D. Appendix A

E. Pathology and Laboratory code

Referencing *CPT Assistant*

Reference *CPT Assistant* to answer the following questions. Document the specific newsletter that addresses the question.

1. Refer to note below CPT code 29530. In the Professional Edition of CPT, what does the following note indicate?

    →*CPT Assistant* Feb 96:3, April 02:13

    _____

    _____

2. The surgeon removed three (3) stones from the ureter. Is it appropriate to report code 50945 *(Laparoscopy, surgical; ureterolithotomy)* for each stone removed from the ureter?

    _____

    _____

3. A physician injects Depo-Medrol into L3-4, and L4-5. Subsequently, the physician inserts another set of needles (to the tar points) to complete the nerve block. Marcaine was injected and the needles were removed. Should the coder assign 64475 *(Injection, anesthetic agent and/or steroid, paravertebral facet joint or facet joint nerve; lumbar or sacral, single level)* for each injection?

_____

_____

4. The surgeon removed a non-tunneled central venous access catheter. CPT provides codes for removal of tunneled devices (36589–36590), but the note under code 36590 states, *"Do not report these codes for removal of non-tunneled central venous catheters."* Should the coder assign an unlisted code?

_____

_____

Application of CPT Exercises

Answer the following questions.

1. The physician performs a synovial biopsy of the metacarpophalangeal joint. Using the alphabetic index, what key word(s) lead you to the coding selection? What is the correct code?

_____

_____

2. The surgeon performed a radical resection of a lesion of the back. The malignant neoplasm extended into the soft tissue. Refer to the term "Lesion" in the alphabetic index. What guidance does the alphabetic index provide? What is the correct code?

_____

_____

3. After an injection of Lidocaine, the surgeon performed a percutaneous tenotomy (Achilles tendon). Refer to 27605–27606. What is the correct code assignment?

_____

_____

4. Using cryosurgery, the surgeon removed four (4) dermatofibromas of the leg. Refer to CPT codes 17000–17250. What is the correct code assignment?

_____

_____

5. Refer to codes 57550–57556. The surgeon performed an excision of a cervical stump, vaginally, with repair of an enterocele. What is the correct code assignment?

_____

_____

Assign CPT codes for the following:

6. Insertion of a Foley catheter (temporary)

_____

_____

7. Biopsy of lacrimal sac

_____

_____

8. Incision and drainage, hematoma, sublingual, masticator space

_____

_____

Chapter 3

Modifiers

Matching

Match the modifier with the correct description.

1. ____ 3P   A. Physical status (anesthesia) modifier

2. ____ F4   B. HCPCS National modifier

3. ____ 73   C. Category II modifier

4. ____ P5   D. CPT Modifier Approved for Hospital Outpatient Use only

5. ____ 53   E. CPT Modifier not Approved for Hospital Outpatient Use

Select the Modifier Exercise

Read the following case scenarios, and indicate the appropriate modifier.

1. A patient seen in the physician's office for his yearly physical (CPT code 99395—*Preventive Medicine E/M*). During the exam, the patient requests that the physician remove a mole on his shoulder. What CPT modifier would be appended to the 99395 to explain that the E/M service was unrelated to excision of the mole?

   Answer: _____

2. A patient is seen in a radiology clinic for an X-ray of the arm (73090). The films were sent to another radiologist (not affiliated with the clinic) to interpret and write the report. What HCPCS Level II modifier would be appended to the CPT code for the services of the radiology clinic?

   Answer: _____

3. A surgeon performed an esophageal dilation (43453) on a 4-week-old newborn who weighed 3.1 kg. What CPT modifier would be appended to CPT code to describe this special circumstance?

   Answer: _____

4. A surgeon performed a tenolysis, extensor tendon of the right index finger (26445). What HCPCS Level II modifier should be appended to the CPT code?

   Answer: _____

5. A planned arthroscopic meniscectomy of knee was planned for a patient. During the procedure, the scope was inserted, but the patient went into respiratory distress and the procedure was terminated. What CPT modifier would be appended to the CPT code (29880) for the physician's services?

   Answer: _____

Coding/Modifier Exercise

Assign CPT codes with the appropriate modifier for the following:

Case Study #1

A surgeon performed a carpal tunnel release (median nerve) on the left and right wrist.

   Index: _____

   Code(s): _____

Case Study #2

A 45-year-old male was brought to the endoscopy suite for diagnostic EGD. Patient was prepped. After moving the patient to the procedure room, and prior to initiation of sedation, he develops significant hypotension, and the physician cancels the procedure. Code for hospital services.

   Index: _____

   Code(s): _____

Case Study #3

A surgeon performed a tonsillectomy and adenoidectomy on a 25-year-old male. Four hours after leaving the surgery center, the patient presents to the clinic with a 1-hour history of bleeding in the throat. The bleeding site was located, however, it was in a location that could not be treated outside the OR. The patient was taken back to the OR for control of postoperative bleeding.

   Index: _____

   Code(s): _____

Case Study #4

Patient presented for capsule endoscopy of the GI tract. The ileum was not visualized.

   Index: _____

   Code(s): _____

Chapter 4
Surgery: Part I

Integumentary System Exercises

Medical Terminology Review

Match the medical terms with the definitions.

1. ____ biopsy   A. freeze tissue

2. ____ basal cell carcinoma   B. removal of damaged tissue from wound

3. ____ cryosurgery   C. removal of a piece of tissue for examination

4. ____ debridement   D. malignant neoplasm

5. ____ lipoma   E. benign neoplasm

Case Studies

Review the documentation and underline key term(s). Identify the terms used to look up the code selection in the Alphabetic Index. Assign CPT codes to the following cases. If applicable, append CPT/HCPCS Level II modifiers.

Case Study #1

With the use of a YAG laser, the surgeon removed a 2.0 cm Giant congenital melanocytic nevus of the leg. Pathology confirmed that the lesion was premalignant.

Index:_____

Code(s): _____

Case Study #2

Operative Note: After local anesthesia was administered, the site was cleansed and an incision is made in the center of the sebaceous cyst. The cyst is drained and irrigated with a sterile solution. Diagnosis: sebaceous cyst of back.

Index: _____

Code(s): _____

Case Study #3

A surgeon reports that the patient has a 2.0 cm basal cell carcinoma of the chin. The excision required removal of 0.5 cm margins around the lesion.

Index: _____

Code(s): _____

Case Study #4

A physician performs a simple avulsion of the nail plate, second and third digits of the left foot.

Index: _____

Code(s): _____

Case Study #5

Operative Procedure: Shaving of a 0.5 cm pyogenic granuloma of the neck

Index: _____

Code(s): _____

Case Study #6

A patient is seen in the Emergency Department after an accident. A 3.0 cm wound of the upper arm required a layered closure and a 1.0 cm superficial laceration of the left cheek was repaired.

Index: _____

Code(s): _____

Case Study #7

Operative Note: Patient seeking treatment for a cyst of left breast. A 21-gauge needle was inserted into the cyst. The white, cystic fluid was aspirated and the needle withdrawn. Pressure was applied to the wound and the site covered with a bandage.

Index: _____

Code(s): _____

Case Study #8

The surgeon fulgurates a .5 cm superficial basal cell carcinoma of the back.

Index: _____

Code(s): _____

Case Study #9

Operative Note: This 59-year-old male developed a sebaceous cyst on his right upper back. After ensuring a comfortable position, the skin surrounding the cyst was infiltrated with $\frac{1}{2}$% Xylocaine with epinephrine to achieve local anesthesia. An elliptical incision surrounding the cyst was made; total excised diameter of 5.0 cm. The cyst wall was dissected free from the surrounding tissues. Hemostatis was obtained and the wound was copiously irrigated. The wound was closed with 3-0 Vicryl, figure-of-eight stitches.

✒ Abstract from Documentation:

What type of lesion was removed? Benign or malignant?

How was it removed?

What is the excised diameter of the lesion?

Did the physician close the wound routinely, or was there a layered closure?

⏱ Time to Code:

Index: _____

Coding Assignment: _____

Case Study #10

Operative Report

Preoperative Diagnosis: 1.0 cm malignant melanoma, right heel

Postoperative Diagnosis: Same

Operation: Wide local excision with split thickness skin graft from the left thigh

Anesthesia: Spinal

Indications: This 72-year old patient has a 1.0 cm malignant lesion of the left heel. He has agreed to a wide local excision.

Procedure: The patient was taken to the operating room, prepped and draped in the usual sterile fashion. A 1/20 of an inch thick split-thickness skin graft (7 cm × 7 cm) was harvested from the left thigh and preserved. Next, the lesion, which was on the medial aspect of the right heel, was excised with 2.5 cm margins down to and including some of the plantar fascia. Total excised diameter was 6.0 cm. Hemostatis was achieved with 2-0 Tycron sutures and the cautery. After suitable hemostasis was obtained, the wound margins were advanced with interrupted sutures of 2-0 chromic and then the skin graft was placed.

The skin graft was approximated to the skin using interrupted running sutures of 4-0 chromic, and then holes were punched in the skin graft to permit egress of serous fluid. Then, a bolster dressing of cotton batting wrapped in Owen's gauze was placed over the skin graft site, and secured to the skin with multiple sutures tied over it to 2-0 Tycron. The skin graft donor site was wrapped with Owen's gauze, two moistened ABD pads and wrapped with a Kerlix and an Ace wrap. The patient tolerated the procedure well and was transported awake and alert to the recovery room in excellent condition.

Abstract from Documentation:

What procedure was performed?

What are the excised diameter, location and type (malignant/benign) of lesion?

What is the coding guideline for coding excision of lesion with subsequent skin replacement surgery? Do you code both or just the skin graft?

What type of skin graft was performed? Adjacent? Skin replacement? Autograft? Cultured tissue?

Was the skin graft full-thickness or split-thickness?

For coding purposes, identify site of defect, size and type of graft:

Time to Code:

Index for Excision of Lesion: _____

Index for Skin Graft: _____

Code Assignment: _____

Musculoskeletal System Exercises

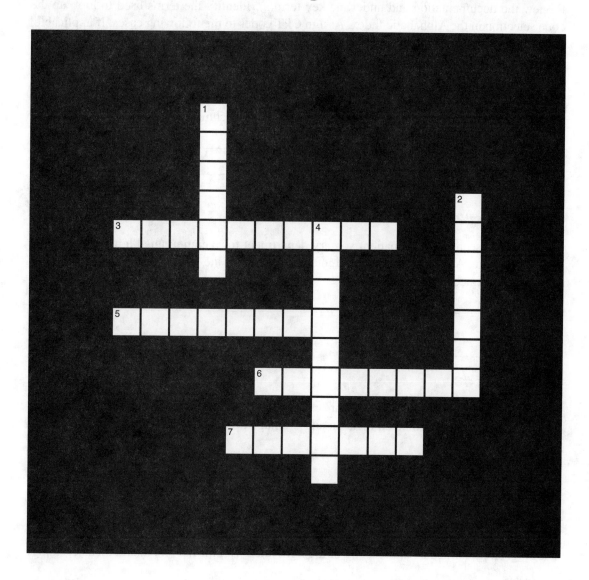

Across

3. Bones of hand
5. Near center of body
6. Cartilage in knee joint
7. Knee bone

Down

1. Away from center of body
2. Bone of upper arm
4. Bones of fingers or toes

Case Studies

Review the documentation and underline key term(s). Identify the terms used to look up the code selection in the Alphabetic Index. Assign CPT codes to the following cases. If applicable, append CPT modifiers.

Case Study #1

The surgeon performed a closed reduction of a scapular fracture.

Index: _____

Code(s): _____

Case Study #2

The patient is seen in the outpatient surgery department for a comminuted left supracondylar femoral fracture. An open reduction and internal fixation of the left supracondylar femur fracture was performed.

Index: _____

Code(s): _____

Case Study #3

The patient had been diagnosed with an infected abscess extending below the fascia of the knee. The surgeon performed an incision and drainage of the abscess.

Index: _____

Code(s): _____

Case Study #4

The surgeon performed an arthroscopy of the right knee with medial and lateral meniscectomy.

Index: _____

Code(s): _____

Case Study #5

The surgeon performed a percutaneous tenotomy of the left hand, second digit and third digit.

Index: _____

Code(s): _____

Case Study #6

Surgeon performed an arthroscopy of the right knee, with limited synovectomy and shaving of articular cartilage.

Index: _____

Code(s): _____

Case Study #7

A patient is diagnosed with osteochondroma of the scapula. The surgeon excises the tumor.

Abstract from Documentation:

What is an osteochondroma?

Time to Code:

Index: _____

Code(s): _____

Case Study #8

Emergency Department Report

Chief Complaint: Left wrist injury

History of Present Illness: The patient is a 5-year-old female that presents in the ED after accidentally falling off her bicycle. She tried to brace her fall with her left wrist and now says there is pain that increases with movement. She had no other injuries, There were no head injuries.

Vital Signs: Blood pressure 117/72, temperature 97.8, pulse 106, respirations 20.

General: The patient is alert, oriented × 3 in no acute distress seated in the hospital bed.

Extremities: Physical exam of the left upper extremity reveals no deformity. To palpation the patient has tenderness of the distal radius and ulna. No tenderness to palpation of the hand. Range of motion is limited in the wrist but intact in the hand and elbow with no tenderness in the elbow.

Emergency Department Course: X-ray of the left wrist revealed a Buckle fracture of the distal radius and ulna. Volar splint and sling were applied. The patient was discharged.

Assessment: Buckle fracture left distal radius and ulna

Plan: Ice and elevate, return if worse, follow-up with orthopedics in 2–3 days, Tylenol with codeine elixir p.r.n. for pain was prescribed.

Abstract from Documentation:

What was the treatment for the fracture?

Time to Code:

Index: _____

Code(s): _____

Case Study #9

Operative Report

Preoperative Diagnosis: Right arm mass

Postoperative Diagnosis: Right arm mass

Procedure: Excision, right arm mass

Indications: This is a 42-year-old woman who presents with palpable enlarging uncomfortable mass in the right upper arm. After discussion, she agreed with excision of the area.

Anesthesia: Local with 1% plain Lidocaine and sedation

Blood Loss: Minimal

Details of Procedure: After informed consent was obtained, the patient was taken to the operating room and placed on the table in supine position. Sedation was administered and the right arm was prepped with Betadine solution and draped sterilely. The palpable mass was identified and an elliptical skin incision was created over the mass along its axis and the underlying mass was excised in its entirety to the level of muscle fascia. It appeared to be most consistent with being multi-lobulated lipoma. It was forwarded to Pathology. The wound was inspected for hemostasis, which was excellent. The deep tissues were approximated with interrupted 3-0 Vicryl and running 4-0 Monocryl subcuticular stitch was used to approximate the skin edges. Benzoin, Steri-Strips and sterile dressing were applied. She was awakened from sedation and returned to the recovery room in stable condition having tolerated the procedure well.

Pathology Report

Final Diagnosis: Soft tissue mass of right upper arm. Lipoma

Gross Description: Received in formalin labeled "lipoma of right arm" consists of a 7 × 4 × 2.5 cm yellow lobulated encapsulated portion of adipose tissue with an overlying 4 × 1.5 cm strip of tan heavily wrinkled unremarkable skin.

✎ Abstract from Documentation:

What was the final diagnosis from the pathologist?

How deep did the mass extend?

What was the treatment for the mass?

Is this a removal of a skin tumor or did it extend into the musculoskeletal area?

⏱ Time to Code:

Index: _____

Code(s): _____

Case Study #10

Operative Report

Preoperative Diagnosis: Mechanical complication from internal 0.062 K wire, first metatarsal, right foot

Postoperative Diagnosis: Same

Procedure: Removal of K wire, right foot

The patient was brought to the operating room and placed on the table in supine position under the influence of IV sedation. Local anesthesia was administered. The right foot was prepped and draped in the usual sterile fashion. The right foot was exsanguinated with an Esmarch bandage and his ankle tourniquet was inflated. A 1 cm dorsal medial skin incision was made directly over the palpable head of the pin. The incision was deepened bluntly, taking care to preserve and retract neurovascular structures. The periosteum was sharply incised from the underlying pin, and the pin was removed with a large straight hemostat. The wound was flushed with copious amounts of sterile normal saline. The skin was reapproximated with a 5-0 Vicryl in a subcuticular fashion. The site was dressed with Xeroform gauze and a dry sterile compression dressing. 4 cc of 0.5% Marcaine was injected for postoperative anesthesia.

✒ Abstract from Documentation:

What is a K wire?

What procedure was performed for this patient?

⏱ Time to Code:

Index: _____

Code(s): _____

Respiratory System Exercises

Medical Terminology Review

Match the following terms with the correct definition.

1. ____ larynx   A. major air passages of lungs

2. ____ esophagus   B. connects mouth to esophagus

3. ____ bronchus   C. structure leads from throat to stomach

4. ____ pharynx   D. a bone in the nose

5. ____ ethmoid   E. voicebox

Case Studies

Review the documentation and underline key term(s). Identify the terms used to look up the code selection in the Alphabetic Index. Assign CPT codes to the following cases. If applicable, assign CPT/HCPCS Level II modifiers.

Case Study #1

The surgeon performed a thoracoscopy for a wedge resection of the lung.

Index:_____

Code(s): _____

Case Study #2

Bronchoscopy with multiple transbronchial lung biopsies taken of the right upper lobe.

Index:_____

Code(s): _____

Case Study #3

A patient seen in the Emergency Department for epistaxis. Physician performs an anterior packing of left nasal passage.

Index:_____

Code(s): _____

Case Study #4

A physician performs a bilateral nasal endoscopy with total ethmoidectomy.

Index:_____

Code(s): _____

Case Study #5

A patient is seen with difficulty breathing due to deviated nasal septum. The surgeon performs a submucous resection of the septum.

Index:_____

Code(s): _____

Case Study #6

The surgeon performs a thoracentesis by placing a needle through the chest wall into pleura to withdraw fluid, which will be sent to the lab for analysis.

Index:_____

Code(s): _____

Case Study #7

A patient was diagnosed with squamous cell carcinoma of the larynx. The surgeon performed a supraglottic laryngectomy with radical neck dissection to remove the metastasis to the lymph nodes.

Index:_____

Code(s): _____

Case Study #8

Operative Report

Preoperative Diagnosis: Chronic laryngitis with polypoid disease

Postoperative Diagnosis: Same

Procedure: Direct laryngoscopy and removal of polyps from both cords

Procedure Detail: After adequate premedication, the patient was taken to the operating room and placed in supine position. The Jako laryngoscope was inserted. There were noted to be large polyps on both vocal cords, essentially obstructing the glottic airway. Using the straight-cup forceps, the polyps were removed from the left cord first. They were removed up to the anterior third, but the anterior tip was not removed on the left side. The polyps were removed from the right cord up to the anterior commissure. There was minimal bleeding noted. The patient was extubated and sent to recovery in good condition.

Abstract from Documentation:

What type of endoscopy was performed?

What procedure was performed during the endoscopy?

Time to Code:

Index:_____

Code(s): _____

Case Study #9

Operative Report

Preoperative Diagnosis: Abnormal chest X-ray and CT scan revealed possible malignant neoplasm of the right upper lobe. Patient is a heavy smoker.

Postoperative Diagnosis: Squamous cell carcinoma, upper right lobe

Procedure: Flexible Bronchoscopy

Procedure: The patient was prepped, draped and after adequate anesthesia, the scope was inserted through the right nares. The scope was advanced further. The vocal cords were normal. Carina was normal. The right main bronchus up into the upper middle and lower lobe bronchi were visualized. The right upper lobe showed an obstructive lesion. Other segments of the middle and lower lobe bronchi were normal. Biopsies and brushings were taken from the right upper lobe bronchus. The patient tolerated the procedure well.

Abstract from Documentation:

What procedures were performed during the endoscopic procedure?

Time to Code:

Index: _____

Code(s): _____

Case Study #10

Operative Report

Preoperative Diagnosis: Bilateral true vocal cord lesions

Postoperative Diagnosis: Bilateral true vocal cord intracordal cyst

Operation: Microlaryngoscopy and biopsy

Indications: This is a 58-year-old man with a history of tobacco use who has had a hoarse voice for the past couple of years. The patient also has an alcohol history. Considering his risk factors and hoarseness, the patient agreed to undergo the surgical procedure to not only better define the lesion but also the nature of the lesion by getting biopsies for pathology.

Operative Findings: Bilateral intracordal mucoid cysts without any evidence of ulcerations or other mass lesions of the vocal cords.

Details of Procedure: Patient was brought to the operating room and laid supine on the operating table. After adequate anesthesia, a Dedo laryngoscope was used to survey the supraglottic area. Once other abnormalities were ruled out, attention was then directed to the true vocal cords. The patient was then suspended using the Dedo laryngoscope and the operating microscope was then brought into the field. Under binocular microscopy the nature of the lesions was better assessed. It appeared that the vocal cords themselves were smooth and very soft to palpation. A boucher retractor was then used to grasp the right true vocal cord and a sickle knife was then used to make an incision laterally. Left-going scissors were then used to create a submucosal flap. The mucoid mass was then extruded and grasped with the non-traumatic graspers and the scissors were then used to dissect the full extent of the mass. The suction was then used to verify the operative site on the right true vocal cord, and once adequate resection was achieved, the mucosal flap was then placed back onto normal position. Attention was then given towards the left intracordal cyst, which was not as prominent as the right.

Again using left nontraumatic graspers the left true vocal cord was grasped and medialized with enough tension so that the sickle knife could be used to make an incision laterally. A submucosal flap was then developed using the suction tip and the mucosal cyst was then identified and carefully excised from the tissues of the true vocal cord, careful not to violate the ligaments or get into the vocals muscle. At this point, once adequate excision was obtained, the mucosal flap was then replaced. At this time, Afrin-soaked pledgets were then used to create adequate hemostasis. The Afrin-soaked pledgets were then removed at the conclusion of the operation. The operating microscope was then taken out the field. The patient was then taken out of suspension and his care was then handed over to the anesthesiologist.

✏ Abstract from Documentation:

What type of endoscopy was performed?

What was performed during the endoscopic procedure?

🕐 Time to Code:

Index: _____

Code(s): _____

Cardiovascular System Exercises

Medical Terminology Review

Match the following terms with the correct definition.

1. ____ fistula   A. surgically closing off a vessel

2. ____ graft   B. blood clot

3. ____ stenosis   C. surgically made passage

4. ____ thrombus   D. piece of tissue that is transplanted surgically

5. ____ ligation   E. narrowing of a passage

Case Studies

Review the documentation and underline key term(s). Identify the terms used to look up the code selection in the Alphabetic Index. Assign CPT codes to the following cases. If applicable, append CPT/HCPCS Level II modifiers.

Case Study #1

A surgeon performed a quadruple coronary artery bypass using a saphenous vein.

Index: _____

Code(s): _____

Case Study #2

Operative Note

Diagnosis: End-stage renal disease

Procedure: Creation of left forearm arterial venous fistula

The patient was prepped and draped in the usual manner. An incision was made over the radial artery and cephalic vein. Each was dissected free to create an anastomosis.

Index: _____

Code(s): _____

Case Study #3

Operative Note

Diagnosis: Thrombosis of right AV (Gore-Tex) graft

Procedure: A transverse incision was made in order to complete a thrombectomy of the graft. Because the balloon catheter could not be passed, it was elected to perform an arteriotomy for removal of the thrombus. The area was irrigated and the incision was closed.

Index: _____

Code(s): _____

Case Study #4

A patient with a previously implanted pacing cardioverter-defibrillator now requires repositioning of the device.

Index: _____

Code(s): _____

Case Study #5

A surgeon performs a percutaneous transluminal angioplasty on the femoral-popliteal artery for a patient with coronary artery disease.

Index: _____

Code(s): _____

Case Study #6

A surgeon performs an axillary-brachial thromboendarterectomy with patch graft

Index: _____

Code(s): _____

Case Study #7

Operative Note

Procedure: Permanent pacemaker implantation.

Details of Procedure: The patient was prepped and draped in the usual sterile fashion. The left subclavian vein was accessed and the guidewire was placed in position. A deep subcutaneous pacemaker pocket was created using the blunt dissection technique. A French 7 introducer sheath was advanced over the guidewire and the guidewire was removed. A bipolar endocardial lead model was advanced under fluoroscopic guidance and tip of pacemaker lead was positioned in the right ventricular apex.

Next, the French-9.5 introducer sheath was advanced over a separate guidewire under fluoroscopic guidance and the guidewire was removed.

Through this sheath, a bipolar atrial screw-in lead was positioned in the right atrial appendage and the lead was screwed in.

🖋 Abstract from Documentation:

What is the coding selection for a permanent pacemaker?

What documentation determines the correct code selection?

🕐 Time to Code:

Index: _____

Code(s): _____

Case Study #8

With an incision into the arm, the surgeon repaired a ruptured false aneurysm of axillary-brachial artery.

Index: _____

Code(s): _____

Case Study #9

Operative Report

Preoperative Diagnosis: Severe left common iliac artery stenosis with claudication

Postoperative Diagnosis: Same

Procedure: Angioplasty of left common iliac artery stenosis

Through a left groin, a 7 French Cordis introducer was placed after the lesion had been crossed with the guidewire. A 9 mm × 4 cm balloon was then chosen. The patient was given 2,000 units of heparin intra-arterially. The balloon was then positioned in the proper location and gently inflated. The stenosis dilated easily. The balloon was inflated for one minute and then brought down. The catheter was advanced, the guidewire removed and completion angiography revealed satisfactory dilatation with no stenosis. The patient was taken to the recovery room in satisfactory condition

✎ Abstract from Documentation:

What main procedure was performed?

What was technique was used to eliminate the stenosis?

🕐 Time to Code:

Index: _____

Code(s): _____

Case Study #10

Operative Report

Preoperative Diagnosis: Status post Port-a-Cath

Postoperative Diagnosis: Same

Procedure: Removal of Port-a-Cath

Indications: The patient has completed the chemotherapy treatment and elects to remove the Port-a-Cath.

Procedure: The patient was placed in supine position. Right subclavian area was prepped and adequately draped. Local anesthesia was given just over the port, and transverse incision was made. Skin incision was deepened down to port area. Fibrinous capsule was exposed and retracted and sharply dissected to remove the soft tissue. Entire fibrinous capsule was excised and then the tunnel was clamped and tied off the fibrinous capsule, after the entire system was removed. The area was irrigated. Hemostasis was assured. Subcutaneous layer was closed using 4-0. Skin was approximated using 5-0 Vicryl running stitches. Steri-strips applied. Patient tolerated the procedure well.

✎ Abstract from Documentation:

What is a Port-a-Cath?

What was the operative action?

🕐 Time to Code:

Index: _____

Code(s): _____

Digestive System Exercises

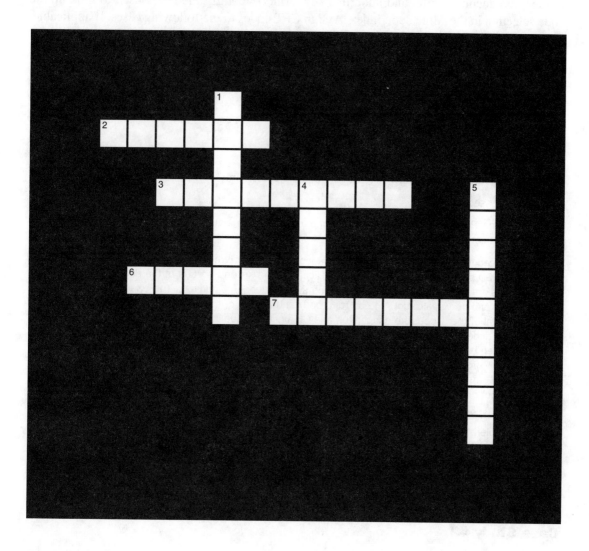

Across

2. Final section of large intestine
3. Instrument to view inside body
6. Third portion of small intestines
7. Groin

Down

1. First part of small intestine
4. From cecum to rectum
5. Navel

Case Studies

Review the documentation and underline key term(s). Identify the terms used to look up the code selection in the Alphabetic Index. Assign CPT codes to the following cases. If applicable, append CPT/HCPCS Level II modifiers.

Case Study #1

Operative Report

Preoperative Diagnosis: Inadequate p.o. intake.

Postoperative Diagnosis: Same

Operation: Percutaneous endoscopic gastrostomy tube placement.

Anesthesia: IV sedation.

Clinical History: The patient is a 75-year-old female patient with inadequate p.o. intake who presents now for PEG tube placement.

Operative Procedure: After establishment of an adequate level of IV sedation and viscous spray of the oropharynx, EGD scope was inserted without difficulty to the second portion of the duodenum from whence it was gradually withdrawn. There were no striking duodenal findings. The pylorus appeared unremarkable and on visualization, the antrum, body and fundus of the stomach were also unremarkable. With withdrawal of the scope, the esophagus and GE junction visualized normal. Insufflation of the stomach was undertaken and at point of maximal transillumination in the epigastrium, local infiltration was undertaken by Dr. June and a slit incision was made. Needle within a cannula was then threaded percutaneously directly into the stomach under visualization. Inner cannula was removed and guidewire was passed. Loop forceps were then passed endoscopically and guidewire was grasped in the stomach and brought out orally, whence it was anchored to a PEG tube which was pulled to emanate via the anterior abdominal wall being anchored to appropriate position.

The patient tolerated the procedure well. There were no complications.

Index: _____

Code(s): _____

Case Study #2

Operative Note: The patient is morbidly obese with a BMI of 37. Procedure performed: Laparoscopic insertion of gastric band.

Index: _____

Code(s): _____

Case Study #3

Diagnosis: Esophageal stricture

Procedure: Upper endoscopy with esophageal dilation

Indications for Procedure: The patient is a 65-year-old woman who has a known esophageal stricture that has required periodic dilation in the past. She has recently had recurrent difficulty with solid food.

Operative Procedure: The instrument was passed easily into the esophagus. The esophagus had normal mucosa. The gastroesophageal junction was present at 30 cm where there was a stricture present and extended for no more than a couple of millimeters in length.

There was a single linear erosion extending about 1 cm above, consistent with reflux esophagitis. Below the stricture, there was a 4-cm sliding hiatal hernia. On retroversion, no additional abnormalities were noted. The body of the stomach distended well and had a normal rugal pattern. The antrum was briefly seen and was normal, as were the duodenal bulb and descending duodenum.

The instrument was withdrawn into the stomach, and a Savary guidewire was passed under direct vision with fluoroscopic control. The instrument was withdrawn, and the patient was dilated with the passage of the 15-, 17-, and 20-mm Savary dilators with minimal resistance encountered and no heme on the dilators.

✎ Abstract from Documentation:

What exactly was visualized during this endoscopic procedure?

Besides visualization (diagnostic endoscopy), what else was performed during the endoscopy?

🕐 Time to Code:

Index: _____

Code(s): _____

Case Study #4

Operative Report

Operation: Ventral hernia repair with mesh Marlex.

History: This is a 45-year-old white male who came in complaining of a bulging mass in the right side of the abdomen. He is a surgical candidate for an initial hernia repair.

Operative Technique: Under general anesthesia, the patient was prepped and draped in the usual fashion. A midline incision from the xiphoid to the suprapubic area was carried out. A lateral flap was developed on the right side as well as the left side. The umbilicus was isolated with an elliptical incision. After completion of the flap and identification of the fascia, there was found a big gap in the midline as well as in the right side of the abdomen. At this point, we proceeded to perform plication of the rectus abdominis muscle. Subsequent to that, we applied the mesh Marlex around the area. Next, we left two Jackson-Pratt drains in the subcutaneous tissue. The redundant skin was resected, and the umbilicus was closed in this area. To close the abdominal wall, we used staples, and for the periumbilical area we used interrupted nylon 3-0. Bleeding was minimal. Condition was good. The patient tolerated the procedure very well and left the operating room in good and stable condition.

✎ Abstract from Documentation:

What is a ventral hernia?

What are the coding guidelines for assigning the implantation of mesh code with a hernia repair?

🕐 Time to Code:

Index: _____

Code(s): _____

Case Study #5

Emergency Department Record

Chief Complaint: Foreign body in throat

History of Present Illness: This is a 73-year-old male who has a history of esophageal stricture, who has had multiple endoscopies to have foreign bodies removed. He was eating roast beef last night and it stuck in his throat. He says anything he tries to eat or drink comes right back up. He called Dr. Ida early this morning and stated that he would meet him in the emergency room. Patient denies any chest pain, fever, chills, shortness of breath or other systemic complaints.

Dr. Ida did an endoscopy and removed several pieces of meat as well as a pea. The patient did receive conscious sedation for the procedure. We watched him in the emergency room on his recovery.

Impressions: Meat impaction in esophagus.

Index:_____

Code(s): _____

Case Study #6

Operative Note

Procedure: Colonoscopy with biopsy

Indications: This 26-year-old female was referred for evaluation because of abdominal pain with occasional episodes of rectal bleeding and some mucus in the stool.

Procedure: The scope was inserted and advanced to the cecum. The rectum showed small pinpoint ulcers but nothing beyond that. I did take some biopsies. The sigmoid colon, descending, transverse and ascending colon was normal.

Index:_____

Code(s): _____

Case Study #7

Operative Report

Preoperative Diagnosis: Thrombosed hemorrhoids

Postoperative Diagnosis: Same.

Indications: This 25-year-old female, one week postpartum, complains of extremely painful hemorrhoids. Examination revealed circumferential prolapsed hemorrhoids with partial thrombosis in multiple areas.

Procedure: After induction of general anesthesia, she was prepped and draped in the usual sterile fashion. The patient was placed in lithotomy position and a retractor was placed in the anus. Very prominent, large, partially thrombosed external hemorrhoid was identified at 7-8 o'clock in the lithotomy position. It was grasped with a hemorrhoidal clamp. A 2-0 chromic stitch was placed at the apex. The Bovie electrocautery was then used to elliptically excise the large hemorrhoid, staying superficial to the sphincter muscle. Bleeding was controlled with Bovie electrocautery. The mucosa was closed with a running chromic stitch, leaving the end-point epidermis open.

Two other very large external hemorrhoids with thrombosis were then identified, at the 5 o'clock position in lithotomy and at the 10-11 o'clock position. These two hemorrhoids were excised in the exact same fashion as the first hemorrhoid. At the conclusion, there was no evidence of bleeding. The patient was returned to the recovery area in good condition.

Abstract from Documentation:

What method was used to remove the hemorrhoids?

Were the hemorrhoids located internally or externally?

Time to Code:

Index: _____

Code(s): _____

Case Study #8

Operative Report

Procedure: Colonoscopy

Indications: Polyp seen on flexible sigmoidoscopy

Procedure: After obtaining consent, the scope as passed under direct vision. Throughout the procedure, the patient's blood pressure, pulse, and oxygen saturations were monitored continuously. The Olympus pediatric colonoscopy was introduced through the anus and advanced to the ileum. The colonoscopy was accomplished without difficulty. The patient tolerated the procedure well

Findings: The terminal ileum was normal. Multiple small-mouthed diverticula were found in the sigmoid colon. A pedunculated polyp was found in the sigmoid colon. The polyp was 30 mm in size. Polypectomy was performed with hot snare after injecting 4cc of epinephrine in the stalk for hemostasis. Resection and retrieval were complete. Estimated blood loss was minimal.

Internal, non-bleeding, mild hemorrhoids were found.

Abstract from Documentation:

Was this a diagnostic or a surgical colonoscopy?

What technique was used to remove the polyp?

Time to Code:

Index: _____

Code(s): _____

Case Study #9

Operative Report

Preoperative Diagnosis: Right colon cancer; probable liver metastasis

Postoperative Diagnosis: Cecal cancer, extensive bilateral liver metastasis

Procedures Performed: Right colectomy and biopsy of right lobe liver nodule

Indications: Patient is a 67-year-old man who presented with anemia. Colonoscopy demonstrated bleeding cecal carcinoma. CT scan suggested liver metastasis. He presents now for a palliative right colectomy and biopsy of liver nodule.

Description: The patient was brought to the operating room and placed in a supine position. Satisfactory general endotracheal anesthesia was achieved. He was prepped and draped exposing the anterior abdomen and a lower midline incision was created sharply through subcutaneous tissues by electrocautery. Linea alba was parted and exploration was performed. The right colon was mobilized by dissection in the avascular plane. The patient had three to four centimeter cecal cancer. The right ureter was identified and preserved.

The terminal ileum and distal ascending colon were divided with GIA-60 stapling devices. The right colic artery and lymph node tissue were resected back to the origin of the superior mesenteric artery with clamps and 3-0 silk ties. The specimen was forwarded to pathology. A stapled functional end-to-end anastomosis was then performed. The antimesenteric edges were reapproximated with a single fire of GIA-60 stapler. The defect created by the stapler was then closed with interrupted 3-0 silk Lembert sutures. The mesocolon was reapproximated with some interrupted 3-0 silk sutures. Hemostasis was confirmed. The right anterior liver nodule was biopsied with a Tru-Cut needle. Hemostasis was achieved. The midline fascia was closed with running 1-0 Prolene suture. The skin was approximated with staples. The wound was dressed. The procedure was concluded. The patient tolerated the procedure well and was taken to recovery in stable condition. Estimated blood loss was less than 100 cc. There were no complications.

Pathology Report

#1-Right Hemicolectomy: Adenocarcinoma of cecum

#2-Liver Biopsies: Metastatic adenocarcinoma

Abstract from Documentation:

Locate the code selection for colectomy. What additional information is needed from the operative report to assign a correct code?

In the index, what code selection is provided for the liver biopsy?

What differentiates between these codes?

Time to Code:

Index: _____

Code(s): _____

Case Study #10

Operative Note

Diagnosis: Gallstone pancreatitis and biliary tree obstruction

Procedure: ERCP

Indications: The patient has gallstone pancreatitis and an ultrasound showed a dilated common duct with stones.

Procedure: an ERCP with sphincterotomy was performed.

Index: _____

Code(s): _____

Chapter 4

Surgery: Part II

Urinary System Exercises

Medical Terminology Review

Match the following terms with the correct definition.

1. ____ -lith   A. sac that stores urine

2. ____ ureter   B. duct leads urine out of body from bladder

3. ____ bladder   C. duct from kidney to bladder

4. ____ kidney   D. stone

5. ____ urethra   E. organ that purifies blood and excretes waste in urine

Case Studies

Review the documentation and underline key term(s). Identify the terms used to look up the code selection in the Alphabetic Index. Assign *surgical* CPT codes to the following cases. If applicable, append CPT/HCPCS Level II modifiers.

Case Study #1

Using calibrated electronic equipment, an uroflowmetry test is performed to measure how well the bladder empties, as well as the storage capacity of the bladder.

Index:_____

Code(s): _____

Case Study #2

Operative Note: Cystoscopy to remove stones from the patient's upper right ureter and another stone lodged in the middle left ureter. Both stones were manipulated back into the kidney with subsequent placement of double J ureteral stents in each ureter.

Index: _____

Code(s): _____

Case Study #3

Operative Note: Patient has a ureteral stricture. Performed a cysto, ureteroscopy and laser treatment of the stricture.

Index: _____

Code(s): _____

Case Study #4

Operative Note: Performed a cystoscopy with resection of a 2.0 cm bladder tumor. The procedure concluded with a steroid injection into the urethral stricture.

Index: _____

Code(s): _____

Case Study #5

Operative Report

Preoperative Diagnosis: History of low grade transitional cell carcinoma

Postoperative Diagnosis: Same

Procedure: Flexible cystoscopy

Indications: Patient is a 49-year-old male diagnosed with low-grade transitional cell carcinoma of the bladder. He is here today for his regular bladder tumor follow-up.

Details: Patient's genitalia were prepped and draped in the typical fashion. 20 cc of 2% lidocaine jelly was instilled into the urethra. The anesthesia was given five minutes to set in. The #19 French flexible cystoscope was passed through the urethra into the bladder. Once inside the bladder, the entire bladder mucosa was evaluated. No lesions were identified. Both ureteral orifices were seen and were found to be normal. At this point, the scope was removed. Patient will be called in three months for his next follow-up.

Index: _____

Code(s): _____

Case Study #6

Operative Report

Preoperative Diagnosis: Multiple bladder stones

Procedure: Cystoscopy with cystolitholapaxy

Indications: This 58-year-old patient was found to have several bladder stones. He is here today for removal of those stones. The patient is voiding well currently. Informed consent was signed and risks and benefits were explained, understood by the patient prior to the procedure. He agreed to proceed.

Description of Procedure: The patient was taken to the cystoscopy suite, placed in dorsal lithotomy position after adequate induction of general anesthesia. Levaquin 500 mg was given intravenously, preoperatively. Perineum and genitalia were prepped and draped in the usual sterile fashion. A #21 French cystourethroscope was inserted into the urethra and the prostate was visualized. He did have some lateral lobe hyperplasia of the prostate, but otherwise no significant pathology in the urethra. The bladder was then entered and drained. Multiple bladder stones were seen and these were all less than half a centimeter apiece. The bladder stones were evacuated using cystoscope and irrigation with the Ellik evacuator. All stones were removed without difficulty. After the bladder was drained and all of the stones removed, the patient was awakened. He returned to the recovery room in satisfactory condition.

Abstract from Documentation:

During the cystoscopy, from which location were the stones removed?

Time to Code:

Index: _____

Code(s): _____

Case Study #7

Operative Report

Preoperative Diagnosis: A 6-mm stone in the left lower pole

Postoperative Diagnosis: A 6-mm stone in the left lower pole

Operation Performed: Left extracorporeal shockwave lithotripsy.

Anesthesia: Intravenous sedation.

Indications for Procedure: This is a 57-year-old man who has been known to have a stone in the left upper pole for a number of years. He recently presented with left renal colic. An X-ray showed the stone to have migrated into the proximal ureter. Recently, he underwent cystoscopy, the stone was successfully flushed into the kidney, and a double-J stent was placed. He now needs to be treated with ESWL.

Description of Procedure: The patient was placed onto the treatment table and, after the administration of intravenous sedation, he was positioned over the shockwave electrode. The X-ray showed the stone to now be located in the lower pole of the left kidney. Biaxial fluoroscopy was utilized to position the stone at the focal point of the shockwave generator. The stone was initially treated at 17 kV, increasing up to 24 kV. The stone was treated with 3000 shocks. Throughout the procedure, fluoroscopic manipulations and adjustments were made in order to maintain the stone in the focal point of the shockwave generator. At the conclusion of the procedure, the stone appeared to have fragmented nicely, and the patient was placed on a stretcher and taken to the recovery room in good condition.

Index: _____

Code(s): _____

Case Study #8

Operative Report

Preoperative Diagnosis: Urethral caruncle
                        Urethral stenosis

Postoperative Diagnosis: Same

Operative Procedure: Cystoscopy
                      External urethroplasty with excision of caruncle

Procedure: The patient is brought to the Cystoscopy Suite where general anesthesia is induced and maintained in the usual fashion. The patient is then placed in the dorsal lithotomy position. The external genitalia are prepped and draped in routine fashion. A 21 French panendoscope is assembled and inserted into the bladder without difficulty. Inspection of the urethra and bladder is carried out with both the straight and the right-angled lenses. The urethra is highly stenotic and it has been difficult to pass the scope, however, it can pop through which caused some bleeding. There is a large caruncle protruding from the urethra, which has been very bothersome for the patient. The urethral mucosa more proximally is normal and bladder neck is normal. The trigone shows significant droppage. The ureteral orifices are identified. The urine efflux is clear from both sides. The orifices are normal in configuration. The remainder of the bladder wall is unremarkable, with no evidence for foreign body of tumor anywhere on the mucosa. Bladder capacity appears about normal.

Following cystoscopy, the urethral caruncle is grasped and then completely excised. An 18 French Foley catheter is inserted into the patient's bladder. Incision into the urethra is made at the 3 o'clock and 9 o'clock positions. Some additional mucosa in the 12 o'clock position is also excised. The Bovie cautery is used to control bleeding. The urethral catheter is removed and inspection reveals that the urethra is somewhat closed and it is necessary to incise the urethra in the 12 o'clock position as well. Once this is done, fulguration controls the bleeding. The catheter is again removed and inspection shows that now the urethra is wide open. There is no significant bleeding. The catheter is reinserted and will be left for drainage for several hours.

Following urethroplasty, the patient undergoes pelvic examination, which is unremarkable. The patient is taken to the recovery room in good condition.

✎ Abstract from Documentation:

What procedures were performed through the endoscope?

In addition to the endoscopy, what other procedures were performed?

⏱ Time to Code:

Index: _____

Code(s): _____

Male Genital System Exercises

Medical Terminology Review

Match the following terms with the correct definition.

1. ____ epididymis   A. organ that produces sperm

2. ____ vas deferens   B. surgical removal of one or both testicles

3. ____ testicles   C. duct that conveys sperm from testicles to urethra

4. ____ orchiectomy   D. surgical removal of foreskin

5. ____ circumcision   E. duct along which sperm passes to vas deferens

Case Studies

Review the documentation and underline key term(s). Identify the terms used to look up the code selection in the Alphabetic Index. Assign *surgical* CPT codes to the following cases. If applicable, append CPT/HCPCS Level II modifiers.

Case Study #1

Patient is a 55-year-old male with a Mentor inflatable three-piece penile prosthesis that had been causing problems. He was experiencing issues with prolonged erections while deflating the prosthesis. It was elected to remove the prosthesis and insert a Duraphase II penile prosthesis. There was some evidence of infection in the area, which was irrigated.

Index:_____

Code(s): _____

Case Study #2

Operative Report

Preoperative Diagnosis: Left hydrocele

Postoperative Diagnosis: Same

Operation Performed: Left hydrocelectomy

Indications: This 55-year-old male with a history of left hydrocele swelling causing discomfort requested intervention after evaluation and preoperative consultation.

Operation: Patient was sterilely prepped and draped in the usual fashion. A transverse incision across the left hemiscrotum was made approximately 4 cm in length down to the level of the hydrocele. Hydrocele was removed from the incision and stripped of its fibrous attachments. Hydrocele was opened and drained. The excess sac was removed and discarded. The sac was then everted with the testicle and a running #2-0 chromic stitch in a locking fashion was placed across the edges of the sac. Meticulous hemostasis was achieved. The testicle and spermatic cord were then replaced back to the patient's left scrotum. There was no damage done to the vas deferens. The dartos layer was reapproximated using #2-0 running locking chromic stitch. The skin was closed in a running horizontal mattress fashion using #3-0 chromic. The patient tolerated the procedure well.

✎ Abstract from Documentation:

Locate hydrocele in the Alphabetic Index. What documentation from the operative report is needed to accurately assign codes?

⏱ Time to Code:

Index: _____

Code(s): _____

Case Study #3

Operative Report

Procedure: Circumcision.

Description of Procedure: The patient was cleaned and draped in sterile fashion and was first numbed at the base of the penis with 1% lidocaine without epinephrine, after which time it was noted that the meatus was at the tip of the penis. The dorsum of the foreskin was then clamped, and an incision was made along the clamp line. The foreskin was then retracted; Gomco bell, size #2, was placed over the tip of the penis, and the foreskin was retracted over the bell and secured with a safety pin. The clamp was then placed and secured. It was held for approximately 5 minutes until appropriate blanching was obtained. The foreskin was then removed with a #11 blade. The Gomco bell and clamp were then removed. There was minimal bleeding. The patient was then dressed with a sterile Vaseline gauze, and the Betadine was also cleaned from the area. He was returned to the newborn nursery, fairly quiet, for observation. The mother was spoken with after the procedure and told that the patient tolerated it well, and she was satisfied.

✎ Abstract from Documentation:

Refer to circumcision in the Alphabetic Index. What information do you need from the operative report to begin your coding assignment selection process?

⏱ Time to Code:

Index: _____

Code(s): _____

Case Study #4

Operative Report

Preoperative Diagnosis: Elevated prostate specific antigen

Postoperative Diagnosis: Same

Procedure Performed: Ultrasound-guided prostate needle biopsy

Anesthesia: General anesthesia

Complications: None

Specimens Removed: Twelve core needle biopsies of the prostate

Indications: The patient is a 57-year-old man. He was found on recent labs to have an elevated PSA at the level of 4.5. He was therefore consented for prostate needle biopsy.

Details of Procedures: Patient was brought back to the Cysto Suite and moved into the lateral decubitus position. After smooth induction of general anesthesia, a digital rectal exam was performed. There were no nodules palpated. The prostate was smooth, firm, and benign feeling. The ultrasound probe was then inserted into the rectum. There were no abnormalities seen on ultrasound. We then proceeded to take a total of 12 core needle specimens of the prostate, two from the right base, two from the right mid, two from the right apex, followed by two from the left base, two from left mid and two from the left apex. The patent tolerated the procedure well. There was minimal blood loss. Patient was transferred back to the Postanesthesia Care Unit in stable condition. He will be sent home with three days of antibiotics and we will follow upon his pathology.

⏱ Time to Code:

Index: _____

Code(s): _____

Case Study #5

Operative Report

Preoperative Diagnosis: T2C, NX, M0 prostate cancer

Postoperative Diagnosis: T2C, NX, M0 prostate cancer

Operation: Radical retropubic prostatectomy with bilateral pelvic lymph node dissection

Indications: This 62-year-old man had an elevated PSA of 12.5 on routine screening. He recently underwent a transrectal ultrasound and biopsy that revealed approximately 9 out of 10 cores positive for adenocarcinoma of the prostate. With hormonal therapy, his PSA preoperatively had decreased to 0.1 on androgen blockade.

Procedure: After administration of general anesthesia, the patient was placed in supine position, prepped, and draped in the usual sterile fashion. A midline incision was made to the left of the umbilicus and carried down to the public bone. The fascia was split in the midline as well as the rectus muscle, and the retropubic space was then entered. Each obturator fossa was delineated using blunt dissection. A fixed Balfour retractor was then placed.

A left pelvic lymph node dissection was then performed in the usual fashion. Care was taken to preserve the obturator nerve. It was noted that there were no grossly enlarged nodes in the area. Clips were used to control bleeding and lymph drainage.

A similar dissection was performed on the right side with no damage to the obturator nerve, and there were no grossly enlarged lymph nodes.

Frozen section analysis did not reveal any adenocarcinoma.

The endopelvic fascia was then identified and defatted. It was split along its lateral borders from the puboprostatic ligaments and down to the bladder neck. The dorsal vein complex and endopelvic fascia were then gathered using a curved Babcock clamp. Two 0 Vicryl suture ligatures were placed at the bladder neck to control bleeding.

A clamp was then passed between the anterior urethra and dorsal vein complex, and a 0 Vicryl suture was then tied around this complex. A second 0 Vicryl suture ligature was also placed in the most distal portion. The dorsal vein complex was divided using electrocautery, and excellent hemostasis was noted. The prostatic apex was identified with further sharp and blunt dissection.

The anterior half of the urethra was divided sharply using the #15 blade. Next, the Foley catheter was passed into the wound and divided. The posterior urethra was then sharply transected in a similar fashion. The catheter was used to provide some subtle traction of the prostate. The rectourethralis was taken down using a right-angle clamp and electrocautery. Each neurovascular bundle was also tied and ligated.

The prostate could be mobilized up to the bladder neck.

The lateral pedicles were controlled using 2-0 Vicryl sutures and divided. A small horizontal incision was then made over the seminal vesicles and ampulla of the vas. Each of these structures was then dissected out using sharp and blunt dissection. Clips were used to control bleeding. The seminal vesicles could be removed in their entirety. Each vas was clipped and ligated.

An anatomic bladder-neck-preserving dissection was then performed, and the prostate was sharply transected off the bladder neck. The bladder mucosa was everted using a running 4-0 Monocryl suture. Two 0 Vicryl sutures were placed at the 6 o'clock position to tighten the bladder neck to 20 French.

Four 2-0 Monocryl sutures were placed in this bladder neck at equally spaced distances. A Greenwald sound was then placed into the distal urethral stump and the corresponding bladder neck sutures were then placed into the urethral stump under direct visualization.

The bladder neck was then brought down to the urethral stump using a curved Babcock clamp. All bleeding was controlled and the wound was irrigated with normal saline. The anastomosis was then tied down and, upon testing, was shown to be watertight.

Two Jackson-Pratt drains were then brought out through each lower abdominal quadrant in a separate stab wound incision. They were used to drain each obturator fossa and around the anastomosis. The fascia was reapproximated using interrupted #1 figure-of-eight Vicryl sutures. The subcutaneous tissue was closed with a running 2-0 chromic suture. The skin was reapproximated using staples. Each drain was sutured in with a 2-0 silk suture. The patient tolerated the procedure well and was discharged to the recovery room in stable condition.

✎ Abstract from Documentation:

Review the Alphabetic Index for the coding selection for Prostatectomy. What documentation would be needed to choose the range to verify?

🕐 Time to Code:

Index: _____

Code(s): _____

Female Genital System Exercises

Medical Terminology Review

Match the following terms with the correct definition.

1. ____ cervix

2. ____ vagina

3. ____ ovary

4. ____ colposcopy

5. ____ laparoscopy

A. surgical procedure; instrument inserted into abdominal wall to view internal organs

B. produces eggs

C. tube leading from genitalia to cervix

D. passage forming lower end of uterus

E. surgical procedure to examine vagina and cervix

Case Studies

Review the documentation and underline key term(s). Identify the terms used to look up the code selection in the Alphabetic Index. Assign *surgical* CPT codes to the following cases. If applicable, append CPT/HCPCS Level II modifiers.

Case Study #1

Operative Note: Patient treated for a 2.5 cm lesion of vagina. The lesion was lasered and hemostasis obtained for bleeding. Specimens sent to pathology for evaluation.

Index: _____

Code(s): _____

Case Study #2

The OB/GYN physician delivers a baby via cesarean section. The physician has provided all obstetrical care prior to delivery and will continue to follow the patient for her postpartum care.

✎ **Abstract from Documentation:**

What coding guidelines pertain to maternity care and are applicable in this case?

🕐 **Time to Code:**

Index: _____

Code(s): _____

Case Study #3

Operative Note: The patient is a 59-year-old Gravida 3, Para 3, who was experiencing postmenopausal bleeding for the last five months and her evaluation included a normal endometrial biopsy. The patient also was found to have a right adnexal mass on CAT scan confirmed with ultrasound as well as a small cystic mass in the left ovary. Given the patient's age and despite a normal CA-125, the need for surgical evaluation of the complex adnexal mass was discussed. The patient also preferred a total abdominal hysterectomy to be performed because of postmenopausal bleeding and to see a definitive diagnosis and treatment of that condition. Informed consent was obtained for hysterectomy and bilateral salpingo-oophorectomy.

Abstract from Documentation:

Review the Alphabetic Index for the selection under the term hysterectomy. What documentation is needed to locate a coding selection?

Time to Code:

Index:_____

Code(s): _____

Case Study #4

Operative Note: This 74-year-old woman underwent a partial vulvectomy 6 months ago for carcinoma in situ. She now was found to have recurrent disease of her vulva and a partial vulvectomy was performed. The skin was dissected towards the introitus and the posterior vagina was dissected for approximately 1 inch into the proximal vagina. The vaginal mucosa was undermined for at least 2 cm and approximated to the perineal skin by interrupted 2-0 Vicryl sutures. The anterior vulva lesion was then excised with a margin of approximately 0.5 cm. The lesion itself was approximately 2 cm in diameter. Bleeding points were cauterized. Wounds closed with interrupted 3-0 Vicryl.

Pathology Report: Specimens: vulva lesion with anal margin, anterior vulva, periurethral

Abstract from Documentation:

Review the Alphabetic Index for coding selections for vulvectomy procedures. What documentation is needed for the coding selection?

Note the definitions for simple, radical, partial and complete vulvectomy codes (listed before code 56405). What documentation from this operative note leads you to the correct definition?

Time to Code:

Index:_____

Code(s): _____

Case Study #5

Operative Note: Patient has chronic complaints of right pelvic pain. Taken to OR for a laparoscopy. Inspection into the pelvis revealed multiple adhesions attached to the left tube and ovary. These adhesions were lysed bluntly with probe. No other abnormalities noted.

Index: _____

Code(s): _____

Case Study #6

Preoperative Diagnosis: Dysfunctional uterine bleeding

Postoperative Diagnosis: Same

Operations: ThermaChoice balloon endometrial ablation

Procedure: The patient was taken to the OR and under adequate anesthesia; she was prepped and draped in the dorsolithotomy position for a vaginal procedure. The Therma-Choice system was assembled and primed. The catheter with the balloon was placed inside the endometrial cavity and slowly filled with fluid until it stabilized at a pressure of approximately 175 to 180 mm Hg. The system was then preheated and after preheating to 87 degrees C, eight minutes of therapeutic heat was applied to the lining of the endometrium. The fluid was allowed to drain from the balloon and the system was removed. The procedure was discontinued.

Index: _____

Code(s): _____

Case Study #7

Operative Report

Preoperative Diagnosis: Perimenopausal bleeding. Possible endometrial hypoplasia

Postoperative Diagnosis: Perimenopausal bleeding

Procedures: Hysteroscopy. Dilatation and curettage

Specimen to Lab: Endometrial curetting.

Estimated Bloods Loss: Less than 5 mL

Description of Procedure: The patient was taken to the operating room and under satisfactory general anesthesia was examined and noted to have a normal-size uterus. No adnexal masses was noted. She was prepped and draped in the routine fashion, the speculum placed in the vagina, and the anterior lip of the cervix grasped with a single-tooth tenaculum. The uterus sounded to 8 cm and easily admitted a #21 K-Pratt, so no further dilation was necessary. A 12-degree hysteroscope was placed, using lactated Ringer as the distending medium, and the cervical canal was normal. The cavity revealed just fronds of tissue. There was tissue sticking out that did not have a particularly polypoid appearance. No other lesions could be appreciated that were polypoid. Curettage with a Milan curette and a serrated curette and then polyp forceps being introduced revealed minimal tissue, and 1 piece of tissue of 5 mm that might be consistent with what was seen on previous sonogram. The hysteroscope was then replaced. No other lesions could be appreciated, and the walls appeared smooth. At this time the hysteroscope was removed, and the tenaculum removed. The tenaculum site was touched with silver nitrate. The bleeding was minimal at the end of the procedure. She was taken to the recovery room in satisfactory condition.

✎ Abstract from Documentation:

What procedures were performed?

Refer to coding textbook, what guidelines pertain to this case?

🕐 Time to Code:

Index: _____

Code(s): _____

Case Study #8

Operative Report

Preoperative Diagnosis: Desire for sterilization

Postoperative Diagnosis: Desire for sterilization

Procedure: Postpartum tubal ligation

Procedure in Detail: The patient was taken to the operating room with an IV line in place. She was placed on the operating room table and a 1.5 cm incision was made in the inferior fold of the umbilicus, continued through the subcutaneous tissue, rectus fascia, and parietal peritoneum as the incision was tracked ventrally using Allis clamps. Peritoneum was entered without difficulty. There was no evidence of vessel damage. Retractors were placed in the incision. At first, the left tube was visualized, grasped with a Babcock clamp, and pulled into the operative field. A hemostat was placed in an avascular plane of mesosalpinx, and a segment of tube was isolated and tied off using 2-0 plain gut. The segment was dissected and handed off the field. Pedicles were bovied. No active bleeding was noted. This was repeated on the opposite side.

Fascia and peritoneum were closed together using running continuous interlocking sutures of 0 Vicryl on a cutting needle. The wound was dressed and the patient taken to recovery in good condition.

✎ Abstract from Documentation:

Refer to the key term in the Alphabetic Index. What information is needed to assign a CPT code for this procedure?

🕐 Time to Code:

Index: _____

Code(s): _____

Case Study #9

Operative Report

Preoperative Diagnosis: Uterine fibroids

Postoperative Diagnosis: Multiple uterine fibroids, uterus -250 g, 2 cm right ovarian cyst

Procedure: Laparoscopic-assisted vaginal hysterectomy with bilateral salpingo-oophorectomy

Procedure in Detail: The patient was taken to the operating room and placed in the supine position. After adequate general anesthesia had been obtained, the patient was prepped and draped in the usual fashion for laparoscopic-assisted vaginal hysterectomy. The bladder was drained. A small infraumbilical skin incision was made with the scalpel, and 10 mm laparoscopic sleeve and trocar were introduced without difficulty. The trocar was removed. The laparoscope was placed and 2 L of CO_2 gas was insufflated in the patient's abdomen.

A second incision was made suprapubically and a 12-mm laparoscopic sleeve and trocar were introduced under direct visualization. A 5-mm laparoscopic sleeve and trocar were placed in the left lower quadrant under direct visualization. A manipulator was used to examine the patient's pelvic organs.

There was a small cyst on the right ovary. Both ovaries were free from adhesions. The ureters were free from the operative field. After measuring the ovarian distal pedicles, the endo-GIA staple was placed across each round ligament.

At this time, attention was turned to the vaginal part of the procedure. A weighted speculum was placed in the vagina. The anterior lip of the cervix was grasped with a Lahey tenaculum. Posterior colpotomy incision was made and the posterior peritoneum entered in this fashion. The uterosacral ligaments were bilaterally clamped, cut and Heaney sutured with #1 chromic. The cardinal ligaments were bilaterally clamped, cut and ligated. The anterior vaginal mucosa was then incised with the scalpel, and with sharp and blunt dissection, the bladder was freed from the underlying cervix. The bladder pillars were bilaterally clamped, cut and ligated. The uterine vessels were then bilaterally clamped, cut and ligated. Visualization was difficult because the patient had a very narrow pelvic outlet. In addition, several small fibroids made placement of clamps somewhat difficult. Using the clamp, cut and tie method, after the anterior peritoneum had been entered with scissors, the uterus was then left without vascular supply. The fundus was delivered by flipping the uterus posteriorly; and through an avascular small pedicle, Heaney clamps were placed across; and the uterus was then removed en bloc with the tubes and ovaries attached.

At this point, the remaining Heaney pedicles were ligated with a free-hand suture of 0 chromic. Sponge and instrument counts were correct. Avascular pedicles were inspected and found to be hemostatic. The posterior vaginal cuff was then closed using running interlocking suture of #1 chromic. The anterior peritoneum was then grasped, and using pursestring suture of 0 chromic, the peritoneum was closed. The vaginal cuff was then closed reincorporating the previously tagged uterosacral ligaments into the vaginal cuff through the anterior and posterior vaginal cuff. Another figure-of-eight suture totally closed the cuff. Hemostasis was excellent. Foley was then placed in the patient's bladder and clear urine was noted to be draining. At the point, the laparoscope was placed back through the 10-mm sleeve and the vaginal cuff inspected. A small amount of old blood was suctioned away, but all areas were hemostatic.

The laparoscopic instruments were removed after the excess gas had been allowed to escape. The incisions were closed first with suture of 2-0 Vicryl through the fascia of each incision, and then the skin edges were reapproximated with interrupted sutures of 3-0 plain. Sponge and instrument counts were correct. The patient was awakened from general anesthesia and taken to the recovery room in stable condition.

✒ Abstract from Documentation:

Refer to the key term hysterectomy in the Alphabetic Index. What key documentation is needed to lead to the correct coding range?

🕐 Time to Code:

Index: _____

Code(s): _____

Nervous System Exercises

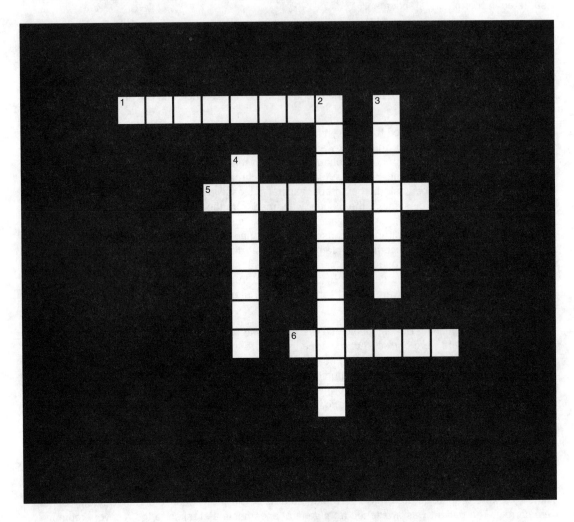

Across

1. Space around dura mater in spinal cord
5. Vertebra of neck
6. Base of spine

Down

2. Surgical removal of vertebrae
3. Major nerve runs back of thigh
4. Tumor of nerves

Case Studies

Review the documentation and underline key term(s). Identify the terms used to look up the code selection in the Alphabetic Index. Assign *surgical* CPT codes to the following cases. If applicable, append CPT/HCPCS Level II modifiers.

Case Study #1

Operative Note for Cervical Epidural Injection: Patient has been experiencing neck pain for several years. Using fluoroscopic guidance, an epidural needle is inserted into the epidural space. A combination of an anesthetic and cortisone steroid solution is injected into the epidural space.

✎ Abstract from Documentation:

Refer to Basic CPT/HCPCS for guidance on coding for spinal injections. What documentation is needed for coding selection?

🕐 Time to Code:

Index:_____

Code(s): _____

Case Study #2

Preoperative Diagnosis: Spinal cord stimulator battery replacement

Postoperative Diagnosis: Spinal cord stimulator battery replacement

Operation Performed: Removal of spinal cord stimulator batteries and replacement with new batteries.

No complications

No specimens

Indications for Surgery: Patient is a 67-year-old man who had spinal cord stimulator implanted approximately five years ago. He comes back because of lack of functioning in this system. Decision was made to proceed with removal of the old batteries and replacement with new one. The patient understands the risks and benefits of the procedure.

Description of Surgery: The patient was placed in supine position and the area where the batteries were located on the left side was prepped and draped in the sterile fashion. The patient was infiltrated with lidocaine 1%. It was reopened with a #15 blade and then the batteries were removed from the pocket and disconnected from the lead wires. A new battery system was reconnected. Wound was closed with #3-0 Vicryl and staples for skin.

✎ Abstract from Documentation:

What is a spinal cord stimulator?

🕐 Time to Code:

Index:_____

Code(s): _____

Case Study #3

Operative Note: Patient has lumbar stenosis at L3-4 and L4-5. Performed a right partial L3 and partial L4 hemilaminectomy with undermining laminotomy for decompression of nerve roots.

Index: _____

Code(s): _____

Case Study #4

Operative Report

Preoperative Diagnosis: Right carpal tunnel syndrome

Operation: Right carpal tunnel release

Indications: The patient is a 55-year-old man who has a history of right hand pain and numbness. He was found to have a right carpal tunnel syndrome by EMG. The patient has been treated conservatively without any improvements, so a decision was made to proceed with a release of the right carpal tunnel.

Description: The patient was placed supine on the operating table, where the right hand was anesthetized with lidocaine 1%. An incision was made with a #15 blade down to the ligament which was incised and was split with sharp scissors. The nerve was found to be completely free. The area was irrigated with antibiotic solution and then the area was closed with #3-0 Vicryl and #4-0 nylon for the skin.

Index: _____

Code(s): _____

Case Study #5

Operative Report

Preoperative Diagnosis: Left ulnar nerve entrapment at the elbow

Postoperative Diagnosis: Same

Procedure: Left ulnar nerve decompression at the elbow

Indications: The patient has a history of numbness in the fourth and fifth digits of the left hand and also some weakness in the grip. He complains of pain in the ulnar side of the left arm. He had an EMG which was positive for entrapment of the left ulnar nerve at the elbow and he had conservation treatment with some improvement of the mode of function, with severe significant numbness and pain. Because of the symptoms, the decision was made to proceed with a decompression of the left ulnar nerve at the elbow.

Description of Surgery: The patient was placed in supine position with the left hand on the surgical stand. The arm was then prepped, draped and then an incision was marked at the level of the left elbow. The incision was infiltrated with lidocaine 1% and then the incision was made with a #15 blade. With the use of bipolar coagulator, the bleeding was easily controlled and then the ulnar nerve was exposed at the level of the elbow proximally and distally. The ulnar nerve was completely compressed, and was released from a dense scar. Antibiotic solution was used to irrigate the area and then the area was closed with #3-0 Vicryl and staples.

Index: _____

Code(s): _____

Case Study #6

Operative Report

Preoperative Diagnosis: Chronic intractable radicular pain

Postoperative Diagnosis: Chronic intractable radicular pain

Procedure: Placement of percutaneous spinal cord stimulator

Indications: This is a 54-year-old man with intractable back and particularly left leg pain for several years.

Details of Procedure: The patient was taken to OR and positioned on his right side. He was prepped with hexachlorophene, and draped using a wound protector. The skin was infiltrated with a mixture of 0.5% Marcaine and 2% lidocaine.

Using a 22-gauge spinal needle, the T12-L1 interspace was sought. After confirming this location on fluoroscopy, the needle was removed; and the Pyle needle was placed. Using radiological images, the Pyle needle was advanced to the epidural space. The Pisces Coag-Plus lead was passed through the needle into the epidural space. Under fluoroscopic guidance, the course of the electrode was monitored as the electrode was passed from the T11-T12 level to the T7 level. At this time, the electrodes were connected, and stimulation was undertaken. Next, the electrodes #2 and #3 were charged, with the #3 electrode getting the negative charge. The patient got excellent coverage of his left leg down below his knee and as far up as his lower back. He was very satisfied with the level and area of coverage. We were able to obtain satisfactory coverage at approximately 3 V with a pulse rate of 50 and a band width of 200. It was decided then to accept this positioning of the electrode, and the electrode was then taped to the patient's back using benzoin and Steri-Strips. Just prior to taping the electrode, the position was confirmed with X-ray. The patient was discharged to the recovery room in satisfactory condition

Index: _____

Code(s): _____

Case Study #7

Operative Report

Preoperative Diagnosis: L5-S1 herniated disc on the left side

Postoperative Diagnosis: L5-S1 herniated disc on the left side

Operation: L5-S1 discectomy and L5 nerve root decompression

Indications for Surgery: The patient is a 53-year-old male who has a history of low back pain and left leg pain in the L5 distribution. An MRI shows the presence of a herniated disc at L5-S1 migrated up impinging the L5 nerve root on the left side. The patient has been treated conservatively without any improvement.

Description of Surgery: The patient was intubated and placed in prone position. Then an incision was marked on the lower back and was prepped and draped in sterile fashion. The incision was made with a #10 scalpel, Bovie coagulator and down to the fascia. At this point, the fascia was incised with a #15 blade. A flap of the fascia was then retracted with #2-0 Vicryl and the muscle was gently dissected and retracted with a Taylor retractor. Under the microscope, a curette was placed between the L5-S1 and X-rays were obtained. The x-rays showed that the curette was between L5 and S1 until under the microscope with microdissection, and with the use of a Midas Rex the lamina of L5 was partially drilled off and yellow ligament was opened, removed and then the L5 nerve root was identified. A large herniated disc was then found, removed and the L5 nerve root was completely decompressed. At this point, the interspace at L5-S1 was entered for the disc removed laterally, and then a complete decompression of the L5 into the foramen was accomplished. At this point, the area was irrigated with antibiotic solution and a paste of Depo-Medrol, Amicar and morphine was left in place. The fascia was closed with a #2-0 Vicryl, subcutaneous tissue with a #3-0 Vicryl, and the skin was closed with subcuticular #4-0 Vicryls.

Abstract from Documentation:

Refer to *Basic CPT/HCPCS Coding* for coding guidance. What is a discectomy?

After the location of the curette was confirmed, what was the first surgical action?

Refer to this term in the Alphabetic Index.

Time to Code:

Index: _____

Code(s): _____

Eye and Ocular Adnexa Exercises

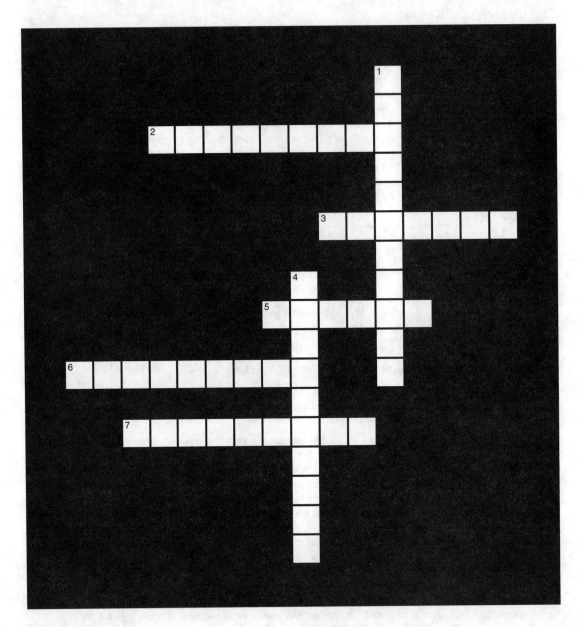

Across

2. Cyst of eyelid
3. Opening of tear duct
5. Drooping of eyelids
6. Eyes deviate outward
7. Benign growth of conjunctiva

Down

1. Inner part of eyelid
4. Abnormal alignment of eyes

Case Studies

Review the documentation and underline key term(s). Identify the terms used to look up the code selection in the Alphabetic Index. Assign *surgical* CPT codes to the following cases. If applicable, append CPT/HCPCS Level II modifiers.

Case Study #1

Patient diagnosed with exotropia. Surgeon performs bilateral recession of lateral rectus muscles.

✎ Abstract from Documentation:

What is the definition of exotropia?

Refer to Basic CPT/HCPCS textbook: How is the lateral rectus muscle classified (vertical or horizontal)?

⏱ Time to Code:

Index:_____

Code(s): _____

Case Study #2

Operative Note: Chalazion incision and drainage of the right eye

Procedure: The right eye was prepped and draped for the procedure. Chalazion forceps were used to grasp the upper eyelid. The surface of the chalazion was incised. The contents of the chalazion were curetted. Chalazion forceps were removed. Hemostasis was achieved. Maxitrol ointment was placed in the eye with an overlying eye pad. The patient was transferred to the recovery area in stable condition.

✎ Abstract from Documentation:

Refer to Chalazion in the Alphabetic Index. What documentation is needed to assign a correct CPT code?

⏱ Time to Code:

Index:_____

Code(s): _____

Case Study #3

Operative Report

Preoperative Diagnosis: Dermatochalasis of bilateral upper eyelids

Postoperative Diagnosis: Dermatochalasis of bilateral upper eyelids

Operation: Bilateral upper lid blepharoplasty

Indications: Patient is a 41-year-old female with a history of progressive upper eyelid hooding related to her redundant skin. The patient complains that this makes her eyelids feel heavy and interferes with her vision, particularly when she is tired. Patient was seen in the Outpatient Clinic and offered bilateral upper lid blepharoplasty.

Details: Patient brought to the operating room and placed on the operating table in supine position. After adequate intravenous sedation had been obtained, the patient's upper eyelids were marked for incision and infiltrated with 5 cc of 0.5% lidocaine mixed with 1:300,000 epinephrine in each lid. The patient's face and head were prepped and draped in the standard operative fashion. The previously marked bilateral upper lids were incised through the skin and the orbicularis muscle using #15 surgical blade. The marked segment was excised sharply with #15 surgical blade with adequate tension on the operative field. The excision was carried down through the muscle and the fat layer was easily visible. This procedure was repeated identically on the opposite lid. Next, the middle fat pad, which was readily identifiable, was gently teased out with a concave applicator and forceps and the pad was removed with the Bovie cautery. Next, the medial fat pad was also dissected out using gentle blunt dissection. The fat pat was retracted into the field and removed using the electrocautery. The procedure was repeated identically on the opposite lid. The operative field was then examined for hemostasis. The electrocautery was used to dry up any small bleeders. The wound was closed in a single layer using interrupted #6-0 Ethibond sutures. The wounds were dressed with Bacitracin and iced moist gauze and the patient was transferred to the recovery room in stable condition.

✐ Abstract from Documentation:

Refer to the key operative term in the Alphabetic Index and note the code range.

What documentation is needed from the record to correctly assign a CPT code(s)?

🕐 Time to Code:

Index: _____

Code(s): _____

Case Study #4

Operative Note: Pterygium removal with conjunctival graft

Procedure Details: Local anesthesia was achieved with a 50/50 mixture of 2% lidocaine and 0.75% bupivacaine with hyaluronidase.. The eye was prepped and draped in the usual sterile fashion. The lashes were isolated on Steri-Strips and the lids separated with the wire speculum. The pterygium was marked with a marking pen and subconjunctival injection of 1% lidocaine with epinephrine was injected underneath the pterygium. The pterygium was then resected and the body of the pterygium was resected with sharp dissection with Westcott scissors. The head of the pterygium was dissected off the cornea with Martinez corneal dissector. The cornea was then smoothed with an ototome bur. Hemostasis was achieved with bipolar cautery.

A conjunctival graft measuring 10 × 8 mm was harvested from the superior bulbar conjunctiva by marking the area, injecting it with subconjunctival 1% lidocaine with epinephrine. This was dissected with Westcott scissors and sutured in place with multiple interrupted 9-0 Dexon sutures. Subconjunctival Dexamethasone and gentamicin injections were given. A bandage contact lens was placed on the eye. Maxitrol ointment was placed on the eye. A patch was placed on the eye. The patient tolerated the procedure well and was taken to the recovery room in good condition.

Index: _____

Code(s): _____

Case Study #5

Operative Note: Patient has possible nasolacrimal duct obstruction.

Procedure: Nasolacrimal duct probing and irrigation for right eye

Procedure Details: The patient was brought into the operating room. The operative eye was prepped and draped. A punctal dilator was used to dilate the superior and inferior puncta of the operative eye. A double-0 Bowman probe was passed through one of the puncta and passed into the common canaliculus. The probe was passed into the nasolacrimal sac and down the bony canal of the nasolacrimal duct. The probe was passed into the nasal cavity beneath the inferior turbinate. The probe was removed. A lacrimal cannula attached to a 3-cc syringe filled with fluorescein solution was used to cannulate the nasolacrimal duct. An aspirating catheter was placed in the ipsilateral nasal cavity. Fluorescein was irrigated into the nasolacrimal duct. Fluorescein was aspirated from the nasal cavity following the irrigation. This demonstrated patency of the nasolacrimal drainage system. The lacrimal cannula and aspiration catheter were removed. The patient tolerated the procedure well and was transferred to the recovery room in stable condition.

Abstract from Documentation:

What documentation is needed to assign the correct CPT code?

Time to Code:

Index: _____

Code(s): _____

Case Study #6

Emergency Department Record

Patient brought to the ED from work with complaints of a foreign body in the right eye. He was wearing safety glasses but stated a piece of metal flew in the eye. He reports slight irritation but no blurred vision. PERLA: Fundi without edema. There was no foreign body on lid eversion. Slit lamp shows a foreign body approximately 2 to 3 o'clock on the edge of the cornea. It appears to be metallic. Iris is intact. There are no cells in the anterior chamber.

Procedure: Two drops of Alcaine were used in the right eye. With use of slit lamp, foreign body was removed without difficulty.

Impression: Residual corneal abrasion

Disposition: Foreign body removed from right eye

Index: _____

Code(s): _____

Auditory System Exercises

Medical Terminology Review

Match the following terms with the correct definition.

1. ____ myringotomy
2. ____ tympanoplasty
3. ____ stapedectomy
4. ____ Eustachian tube
5. ____ tympanum

A. connects middle ear with nasopharynx

B. eardrum

C. surgical incision into eardrum

D. surgical removal of innermost chain of 3 ossicles in middle ear

E. surgical repair of middle ear

Case Studies

Review the documentation and underline key term(s). Identify the terms used to look up the code selection in the Alphabetic Index. Assign *surgical* CPT codes to the following cases. If applicable, append CPT/HCPCS Level II modifiers.

Case Study #1

Physician Office Note: Examination of the ear canal on both sides revealed impacted cerumen, tightly on the right side and a little bit on the left. With the use of ear curet, the impacted cerumen was removed. Both ears were irrigated with saline solution and suctioned dry to clean out all the debris.

Index: _____

Code(s): _____

Case Study #2

Operative Report

Preoperative Diagnosis: Recurrent otitis media with persistent bilateral middle ear effusion

Postoperative Diagnosis: Same

Procedure: Bilateral myringotomy with ventilating tube insertion

Procedure in Detail: The patient was prepped and draped in the usual fashion under general anesthesia. Myringotomy was performed in the anterior-inferior quadrant and thick fluid suctioned from the middle ear space. A Type I Paparella tube was then inserted. Then a myringotomy was performed on the left ear, again thick fluid was suctioned from the middle ear space. A Type I Paparella tube was then inserted. Cortisporin Otic Suspension drops were then placed in both ear canals and cotton in the ears. The patient was awakened and returned to the recovery room in satisfactory condition.

✒ Abstract from Documentation:

Refer to Basic CPT/HCPCS textbook for guidelines pertaining to myringotomy for insertion of tubes.

🕘 Time to Code:

Index:_____

Code(s): _____

Case Study #3

Operative Report

Preoperative Diagnosis: Left tympanic membrane perforation

Postoperative Diagnosis: Left tympanic membrane perforation

Procedure: Left tympanoplasty

Indications for Operation: This patient is a man who sustained a tympanic membrane perforation 20 years ago after diving into a pool. He has now sought repair.

Details of Operation: After induction of anesthesia, the table was rotated 180 degrees and the left ear was prepped and draped in sterile fashion. Operating microscope was then used to inspect the left ear. A large central perforation encompassing approximately 50% of the tympanic membrane was visualized. Malleus was clearly visualized and appeared intact. Using 1% lidocaine with 1:1000 epinephrine injection, four quadrant canal injection was performed. Next, the patient was rotated away and a postauricular incision was made. Temporalis fascia was harvested and kept aside. A T-shaped incision was made on soft tissue and Lempert elevator was used to elevate the canal walls again. A freer was used to elevate the canal walls again and the previously made canal wall incisions were identified. The vascular flap was then raised. Canal wall skin was elevated to the level of the annulus, which was then elevated. The middle ear space was entered through the mucosa using a Rosen. The chorda tympani nerve was identified and preserved. The tympanic membrane was then raised off the chorda tympani nerve and the malleus. Gelfoam was placed in the anterior most aspect of the middle ear space, and the fascia was then laid into place. Tympanic membrane was laid down over the fascia. The vascular flap was then laid back down and the postauricular incision was closed with Vicryl sutures. PSO ointment was applied to the middle ear space and at this point, the left ear was cleaned. Sterile dressing was then placed over the ear and the patient was returned to the recovery room.

✒ Abstract from Documentation:

Refer to tympanoplasty in the Alphabetic Index. What types of documentation should be searched for when reading the operative report?

🕘 Time to Code:

Index:_____

Code(s): _____

Case Study #4

Operative Report

Preoperative Diagnosis: Conductive hearing loss, right ear

Postoperative Diagnosis: Conductive hearing loss, right ear

Operation: Stapedectomy

Procedure: The patient was prepped and draped in the usual manner. The external auditory canal wall was injected with 1% lidocaine and 1:100,000 epinephrine. The tympanomeatal flap was elevated using a vertical rolling knife. The middle ear was entered and chorda tympani nerve identified and annulus lifted out of the tympanic sulcus. After elevating the tympanomeatal flap anteriorly, the ossicles were palpated and the malleus and incus moved freely and the stapes was fixed. The posterior superior canal wall was curetted down after mobilizing the chorda tympani nerve, which was left intact. The stapes footplate was easily visualized and found to be markedly thickened. The pyramidal process was identified and the stapes tendon cut, and an IS joint knife was used to dislocate the joint between the incus and stapes. Next, a small and a large Buckingham mirror were used along with a drill to drill out the stapes footplate. After this was done, a .5 x 4-mm Schukneckt piston prosthesis was placed in position. Crimping was the achieved and there was an excellent fit, and the stapes footplate area was then packed with small pieces of Gelfoam. The tympanomeatal flap was then put back in proper position, and the middle ear was then packed with rayon strips of Cortisporin and a cotton ball in the middle to form a rosette. The patient was awakened in the operating room and transferred to recovery in no apparent distress.

Index: _____

Code(s): _____

Chapter 5

Radiology

Medical Terminology Review

Match the following terms with the correct definition.

1. _____ CT Scan

2. _____ Nuclear Medicine

3. _____ MRI

4. _____ Ultrasound

5. _____ X-ray

A. uses electromagnetic radiation to make images

B. creates multiple images with computer technology to provide cross-sectional views

C. uses powerful magnet and radio waves to take images

D. uses high-frequency sound waves to view organs and structures in body

E. images developed based on energy emitted from radio-active substances

Case Studies

Identify the key term from the index and assign radiology codes to the following cases.

Case Study #1

Radiology Report

Left Ankle (two views): The left ankle shows no evidence of fracture or dislocation. The visualized bones and their respective articular surfaces are intact.

Conclusion: Normal left ankle

Index: _____

Code(s): _____

Case Study #2

X-ray of elbow, 3 views

Radiograph: Left elbow, 3 views

Indications: Pain in elbow after fall

Findings: There is a mildly displaced, slightly angulated fracture involving the supracondylar portion of the distal humerus. There is associated joint effusion reflecting hemarthrosis.

Index: _____

Code(s): _____

Case Study #3

Bilateral Screening Mammogram

Comparison was made to multiple prior studies.

Findings: Examination demonstrates moderately dense fibroglandular tissue. A nodular density is seen in the left central areolar region, which was seen on the prior studies and is essentially unchanged. There is no evidence of any suspicious calcifications. Skin and nipples have no abnormality. As compared with prior study, there is no significant interval change.

Impression: No radiographic evidence of malignancy. No significant interval change since prior study.

Index: _____

Code(s): _____

Case Study #4

CT Scan of the Head

Technique: Non-contrast CT scan of the head

Findings: No evidence of acute bleed is noted. The ventricles are not dilated and are maintained in their midline position. No evidence of any low attenuation area, especially in the basal ganglia or in the brainstem, noted to suggest acute or old infarct. The posterior fossa appears normal. No abnormal calcifications are seen.

Impression: No evidence of acute bleed identified. No midline shift or acute infarct noted.

Index: _____

Code(s): _____

Case Study #5

KUB, Upper GI Series

The KUB study reveals a large amount of fecal matter present in the colon. Staples are seen in the right upper quadrant. The stomach is high and transverse in type. There is a small sliding hiatal hernia and there is small gastroesophageal reflux. The duodenal bulb fills without ulceration. The stomach empties well.

Opinion: Small sliding hiatal hernia with intermittent gastrointestinal reflux

Index: _____

Code(s): _____

Case Study #6

Upper Abdominal Ultrasound

The gall bladder, liver, pancreas, kidneys and spleen are well delineated and appear normal. The bile ducts are not distended. The abdominal aorta and inferior vena cava are normal in caliber.

Opinion: Normal upper abdominal sonogram.

Index: _____

Code(s): _____

Case Study #7

Oral Cholecystogram

The gallbladder concentrates the contrast medium well and numerous radiolucent calculi are demonstrated.

Diagnosis: Cholelithiasis

Index: _____

Code(s): _____

Case Study #8

CT Scan, right elbow

Tomographic cuts were taken through the elbow at 3-mm intervals in AP and lateral views. No bone or joint abnormalities are evident. No fracture is evident.

Impression: Normal right elbow

Index: _____

Code(s): _____

Case Study #9

KUB and Intravenous Pyelogram

The KUB is normal. No urinary calcifications can be identified.

Following the intravenous injection, there is a good delineation of the urinary tract. The kidneys are small, measuring 9.5 cm in their greatest length. The renal collecting system, ureters, and bladder appear normal.

Opinion: The kidneys measure slightly small. The urinary tract is otherwise normal.

Index: _____

Code(s): _____

Case Study #10

Chest X-ray

PA and lateral chest

The cardiopericardial silhouette and mediastinum are within normal limits. There is a left lower lobe infiltrate suspect for pneumonia. In addition, the right cardiac border is ill defined which may represent a right middle lobe infiltrate or atelectasis. There is surgical hardware of the lower cervical spine.

Impression: Left lower lobe infiltrate suspect for pneumonia. Probable right middle lobe infiltrate.

Index: _____

Code(s): _____

Chapter 6

Pathology and Laboratory

Case Studies

Identify the key term from the index and assign pathology and laboratory codes to the following cases.

Case Study #1

GENERAL CHEMISTRY

Sodium	Potassium	Chloride	Total CO_2	Glucose	BUN	Creatinine	Ionized Calcium
138	3.3	96	34	104	20	0.8	6.0

Index:_____

Code(s): _____

Case Study #2

Pathology Report

Specimen: Prostate Chips

Gross Examination: One specimen is received in formalin labeled with demographics and prostate chips. It consists of gray-tan, rubbery fragments of tissue measuring in aggregate 2.9 × 2.5 × 1.5 cm. The specimen is entirely submitted in cassettes A1-A4.

Microscopic Examination: Benign Prostatic Hypertrophy

Index:_____

Code(s): _____

Case Study #3

A stool sample is submitted to the lab for Helicobacter pylori.

Index:_____

Code(s): _____

Case Study #4

A 55-year-old female is seen in the physician's office for an elevated blood pressure. She reports that there is a family history of kidney disease. A Cystatin C test is performed.

Index:_____

Code(s): _____

Case Study #5

A physician suspects that a patient might have an adrenocortical insufficiency and orders an insulin tolerance panel (Cortisol and Glucose) test.

Index:_____

Code(s): _____

Case Study #6

Pathology Report

Specimen: Nasal Cyst

Gross Description: One specimen received in formalin labeled "nasal cyst." Skin measuring 1.7 × 0.8 × 0.5 cm. The specimen is serially sectioned revealing a 0.3 cm in diameter cyst containing white mucous-like material.

Microscopic Description: Skin, nose consistent with sebaceous adenoma

Index:_____

Code(s): _____

Case Study #7

Lipid Panel

Test	Result	Reference Ranges
Cholesterol, serum	206	75–200
HDL	51	30–70
Triglycerides	119	20–250

Index:_____

Code(s): _____

Case Study #8

Urine Culture

Source: Straight Catheter

Abundant Gram Positive Cocci Suggestive of Streptococci

>100,000 CFU/ML Serratia Marcescens

>100,000 CFU/ML Enterococcus Species

Index: _____

Code(s): _____

Case Study #9

Test Name	Glycohemoglobin
Reference Range	3.6–6.8
Result	5.9

Index: _____

Code(s): _____

Case Study #10

An 8-year-old child presents in the urgent care center for abdominal pain associated with some diarrhea. The physician orders a fecal calprotectin test.

Index: _____

Code(s): _____

Chapter 7

E/M

Case Studies

Answer the following questions and/or assign Evaluation and Management codes to the following cases.

Case Study #1

The patient was seen in the physician's office after falling and injuring her ankle. The physician performed a brief HPI, a problem-focused exam and the decision-making was straightforward. What component(s) of the history is missing from this scenario?

Case Study #2

A new patient is seen in the physician's office for dull ache in his left side. The physician performs a detailed history and physical examination and the medical decision-making was of moderate complexity. What is the correct E/M code for this service?

Case Study #3

A 49-year-old established patient visits his family physician for a physical that is required by his place of employment. The physician documents a comprehensive history, exam and orders a series of routine tests such as a chest X-ray and EKG. In addition, the physician counsels the patient about smoking habit. What CPT code would be selected to represent this service?

Case Study #4

The physician documents that the patient has a cough, fever and muscle aches. A review of systems is performed, a detailed account of present illness is documented and the physician outlines the management options, complexity of treatment plan and orders tests. What key E/M component is missing from this documentation?

Case Study #5

A patient is seen on January 23, 2006 by a primary care physician who is a member of University Associates. A cardiologist (also a member of University Associates) sees the patient on November 24, 2007. Would the visit on November 24th be classified as a *new* or an *established* patient?

Case Study #6

An established patient is seen in the physician's office for counseling after having an extremely high cholesterol reading and hypertension. Which range of codes would be used to select the appropriate CPT code for these services?

Case Study #7

The physician sees a patient in Sunny Acres Nursing Facility as a follow-up visit. The patient has a urinary tract infection that is not responding to medication. The physician documents a problem-focused interval history, expanded problem-focused exam and the medical decision-making was of moderate complexity. What is the correct CPT code assignment for this service?

Case Study #8

A patient is seen in the Emergency Department for severe low back pain. The ED physician performs an expanded problem-focused history, problem-focused examination, and the medical decision-making was of moderate complexity. What is the correct E/M code assignment for this service?

Case Study #9

Physician documents that critical care services were provided to a 12-year-old patient for 90 minutes. What is the correct E/M code assignment for this service?

Case Study #10

A 55-year-old patient (post Lasix surgery) visits a new ophthalmologist for extreme dry eyes. The physician performs an expanded problem-focused history and exam and prescribes eye drops as needed. What is the correct E/M code assignment for this service?

Chapter 8

Medicine

Case Studies

Identify the key term from the index and assign codes from the Medicine Section to the following cases.

Case Study #1

A 35-year-old patient receives an IM injection of the Lyme disease vaccine.

    Index: _____

    Code(s): _____

Case Study #2

A 45-year-old patient complains of sneezing, coughing and occasional episodes of wheezing. The physician wants to determine the cause of these allergic symptoms and performs 30 percutaneous skin tests.

    Index: _____

    Code(s): _____

Case Study #3

A 55-year-old patient with Type II diabetes mellitus emails her registered dietitian to ask advice about a adding a food product to her diet. The dietitian promptly responds to the question and keeps a record of this correspondence. The date of the last visit was two weeks ago.

    Index: _____

    Code(s): _____

Case Study #4

A 45-year-old patient with end-stage renal disease (ESRD) is seen in the outpatient dialysis clinic for services on July 2, 5, 9, 15, 18, 21, 24, and 28.

Index: _____

Code(s): _____

Case Study #5

A 59-year-old female is undergoing chemotherapy treatment. She is seen in the clinic for a refill for her portable infusion pump.

Index: _____

Code(s): _____

Case Study #6

A patient is seen in the Emergency Department with severe vomiting and diarrhea due to viral gastroenteritis. IV hydration prescribed and takes one hour to administer.

Index: _____

Code(s): _____

Case Study #7

Patient was diagnosed with actinic keratosis with lesions on several locations of the face. The patient receives irradiation of the areas with photodynamic therapy illuminator for 15 minutes.

Index: _____

Code(s): _____

Case Study #8

A 67-year-old patient with multiple medical problems is currently taking six prescriptions and several over-the-counter agents. The primary care physician has a concern about side effects; therefore; the patient is referred to a pharmacist for assessment and management of medications. The pharmacist assesses the treatment and makes recommendations during the 10 minute face-to-face visit.

Index: _____

Code(s): _____

Case Study #9

A 32-year-old female is referred to the Behavioral Health Clinic due to significant personality changes. A series of tests is administered to evaluate the patient's emotionality, intellectual abilities, personality and psychopathology. The computerized test is completed in order to assist with establishing a diagnosis.

Index: _____

Code(s): _____

Case Study #10

ELECTROENCEPHALOGRAM

Complaint: Altered mental status

Current Medications: Vasotec, Lanoxin and Lasix

State of patient during recording: awake

Description: The background is characterized by diffuse slowing and disorganization consisting of medium-voltage theta rhythm at 4-6 Hz seen from all head areas. From anterior head areas, faster activity at beta range. Eye movements and muscle artifacts are noted. Photic stimulation and hyperventilation were not performed. Total recording time was 40 minutes.

IMPRESSION: This is a moderately abnormal record due to diffuse slowing and disorganization of the background, with the slowing being at theta range.

Index: _____

Code(s): _____

Chapter 9
Anesthesia

Case Studies

Identify the key term from the index and assign anesthesia codes to the following cases:

Case Study #1

Patient admitted for uterine fibroids and dysmenorrhea. The surgeon performs a vaginal hysterectomy.

    Index:_____

    Code(s): _____

Case Study #2

Patient admitted for a right ureteral stent placement. The surgeon performs a cystoscopy with insertion of ureteral stent.

    Index:_____

    Code(s): _____

Case Study #3

This is a 49-year-old man with a chronic right-sided submandibular swelling occurring over the last few years. The diagnosis of right sialoadenitis was made. An excision of right submandibular gland was performed.

    Index:_____

    Code(s): _____

Case Study #4

Patient is being treated for a lateral meniscus tear. The surgeon performs an arthroscopy meniscectomy.

    Index:_____

    Code(s): _____

Case Study #5

The patient is a 65-year-old male who was recently treated for low anterior resection for a stage II superior rectal cancer. Adjuvant chemotherapy is planned. Placement of long-term venous access device was requested. Surgeon inserts a Port-a-Cath.

Index: _____

Code(s): _____

Case Study #6

The patient is a 76-year-old male with substantial underlying pulmonary disease. He has required mechanical ventilation for approximately two to three weeks and failed several attempts to be completely taken off mechanical ventilation. He was brought to the operating room for placement of a tracheostomy tube.

Index: _____

Code(s): _____

Case Study #7

The patient is a 56-year-old male who presented to the ENT Clinic with a history of left-sided nasal obstruction. The following procedures were performed: left maxillary sinusotomy, left anterior ethmoidectomy and removal of left nasal polyposis.

Index: _____

Code(s): _____

Case Study #8

The patient is a 56-year-old man previously diagnosed with pancreatic cancer. The surgeon performs a partial excision of the pancreas.

Index: _____

Code(s): _____

Case Study #9

Patient has a diagnosis of urinary retention. The surgeon performs a transurethral resection of the prostate.

Index: _____

Code(s): _____

Chapter 10

HCPCS

Case Studies

Identify the key term from the index and assign codes from the *HCPCS Level II* to the following cases.

Case Study #1

Clubfoot wedge to modify a shoe

Index: _____

Code(s): _____

Case Study #2

Patient with asthma requires a nebulizer with compressor.

Index: _____

Code(s): _____

Case Study #3

Patient has extreme dry eyes. Physician inserts temporary, absorbable lacrimal duct implants in each eye.

Index: _____

Code(s): _____

Case Study #4

Injection of 50 mg of progesterone

Index: _____

Code(s): _____

Case Study #5

At-risk assessment for patient who is 10 weeks pregnant.

Index: _____

Code(s): _____

Case Study #6

Standard metal bed pan

Index: _____

Code(s): _____

Case Study #7

Screening mammography, bilateral (direct digital image)

Index: _____

Code(s): _____

Case Study #8

Injection 500 mg vancomycin HC1

Index: _____

Code(s): _____

Case Study #9

IV pole for infusion

Index: _____

Code(s): _____

Case Study #10

Arthroscopy of left knee for cartilage debridement of medial compartment and removal of loose bodies in lateral compartment

Index: _____

Code(s): _____

Chapter 11

Reimbursement in the Ambulatory Setting

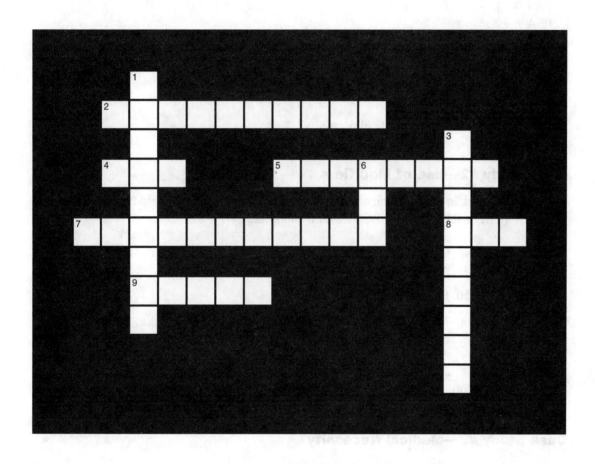

Across

2. Incorrectly assigning multiple codes

4. Develops yearly Workplan

5. Assigning a code for higher payment

7. RVUs include physician work, practice and _____ expenses

8. Reimbursement system for ambulatory surgery centers

9. Reimbursement system for physicians

Down

1. Status indicator X identifies _____ services

3. Status indicator C describes _____ procedures

6. Tool used to weed out incorrect claims

Case Studies

Review the following case studies and answer the questions that follow.

Case Study #1—Medical Necessity

A 47-year-old female patient is seen in an outpatient setting for a variety of symptoms, including: fatigue, weakness and insomnia. The physician orders the following tests:

```
FBS
PSA
WBC
T3, T4
TSH
```

Which test(s) does not meet medical necessity?

Case Study #2—Use of Modifiers

Place a check mark in front of each of the following CPT code(s) that should **NOT** be appended with a LT (left) or RT (right) HCPCS Level II modifier.

1. _____ 28445 Open treatment of talus fracture, includes internal fixation, when performed

2. _____ 28150 Phalangectomy, toe, each toe

3. _____ 11400 Excision, benign lesion including margins, except skin tag (unless listed elsewhere), trunk, arms, or legs; excised diameter 0.5 cm or less

4. _____ 23500 Closed treatment of clavicular fracture; without manipulation

5. _____ 71060 Bronchography, bilateral, radiological supervision and interpretation

Case Study #3—Medical Necessity

Match the following diagnoses/symptoms with the appropriate test/procedure.

1. _____ R/O pregnancy   A. spirometry

2. _____ low back pain   B. EKG

3. _____ hearing loss   C. Human chorionic gonadotropin (hCG)

4. _____ COPD   D. osteopathic manipulative treatment

5. _____ coughing, sneezing, runny nose   E. tympanometry

6. _____ tachycardia   F. allergy tests

Answer Key

Chapter 1
Introduction to Clinical Coding

Case Study #1

The patient is seen as an outpatient for a bilateral mammogram.

CPT Code: 77055–50

Note that the description for code 77055 is for a unilateral (one side) mammogram. 77056 is the correct code for a bilateral mammogram. Use of modifier –50 for bilateral is not appropriate when CPT code descriptions differentiate between unilateral and bilateral.

Case Study #2

Physician performs a closed manipulation of a medial malleolus fracture—left ankle.

CPT Code: 27766–LT

The code represents an open treatment of the fracture, but the physician performed a closed manipulation. Correct code: 27762–LT

Case Study #3

Surgeon performs a cystourethroscopy with dilation of a urethral stricture.

CPT Code: 52341

The documentation states that it was a urethral stricture, but the CPT code identifies treatment of ureteral stricture. Correct code: 52281

Case Study #4

The operative report states that the physician performed Strabismus surgery, requiring resection of the medial rectus muscle.

CPT Code: 67314

The CPT code selection is for resection of one vertical muscle, but the medial rectus muscle is horizontal. Correct code: 67311

Case Study #5

The chiropractor documents that he performed osteopathic manipulation on the neck and back (lumbar/thoracic).

CPT Code: 98925

Note in the paragraph before code 98925, the body regions are identified. The neck would be the cervical region; the thoracic and lumbar regions are identified separately. Therefore, three body regions are identified. Correct code: 98926

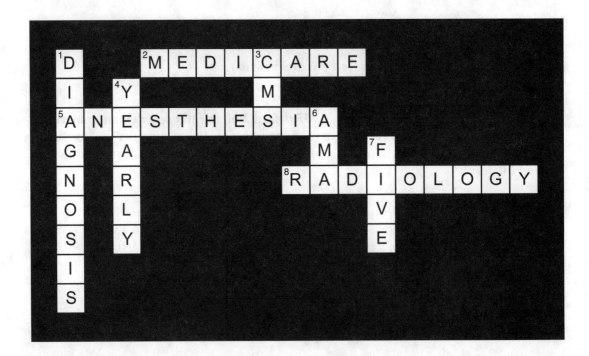

Across

2. Federal insurance for those over age 65 [MEDICARE]

5. Modifier P4 found in this CPT section [ANESTHESIA]

8. CT Scans found in this section of CPT [RADIOLOGY]

Down

1. Supports medical necessity [DIAGNOSIS]

3. Agency administers Medicare [CMS]

4. A new edition of CPT is published _____ [YEARLY]

6. Organization that publishes CPT [AMA]

7. Number of digits in CPT code [FIVE]

Chapter 2
Application of the CPT System

Matching Exercise

1. ____ Complete list of modifiers (D)   A. Appendix B
2. ____ Complete list of add-on codes (C)   B. Category II code
3. ____ 82525 Copper (E)   C. Appendix D
4. ____ Complete list of recent additions,   D. Appendix A
deletions and revisions (A)
E. Pathology and Laboratory code
5. ____ 1039F Intermittent asthma (B)

Referencing *CPT Assistant*

1. Refer to note below CPT code 29530. In the Professional Edition of *CPT Assistant,* what does the following note indicate?

   →*CPT Assistant* Feb 96:3, April 02:13

   This note refers the coder to the February 1996 edition of *CPT Assistant* (page 3) and April 2002 (page 13) for additional information about use of this code.

2. The surgeon removed three (3) stones from the ureter. Is it appropriate to report code 50945 *(Laparoscopy, surgical; ureterolithotomy)* for each stone removed from the ureter?

   Answer: No. Code 50945 is intended to be reported once per surgical session, regardless of the number of stones removed. (*CPT Assistant,* September 2006)

3. A physician injects Depo-Medrol into L3-4, and L4-5. Subsequently, the physician inserts another set of needles (to the tar points) to complete the nerve block. Marcaine was injected and the needles were removed. Should the coder assign 64475 *(Injection, anesthetic agent and/or steroid, paravertebral facet joint or facet joint nerve; lumbar or sacral, single level)* for each injection?

   Answer: No. Code 64475 should be reported only once. (*CPT Assistant,* May 2004)

4. The surgeon removed a non-tunneled central venous access catheter. CPT provides codes for removal of a tunneled devices (36589–36590) but the note under code 36590 states, *"Do not report these codes for removal of non-tunneled central venous catheters."* Should the coder assign an unlisted code?

   Answer: No. The work required for non-tunneled central venous access catheter is considered to be inherent in the evaluation and management visit in which it is performed. (*CPT Assistant,* September 2004)

Application of CPT Exercises

1. The physician performs a synovial biopsy of the metacarpophalangeal joint. Using the Alphabetic Index, what key word(s) lead you to the coding selection? What is the correct code?

   Answer:
   Synovium, Biopsy, Metacarpophalangeal Joint 26105
   Biopsy, Metacarpophalangeal Joint 26105
   Metacarpophalangeal Joint, Biopsy, Synovium 26105

2. The surgeon performed a radical resection of a lesion of the back. The malignant neoplasm extended into the soft tissue. Refer to the term "Lesion" in the alphabetic index. What guidance does the Alphabetic Index provide? What is the correct code?

   Answer: Under the term "Lesion," there is no entry for back. The note under Lesion states to "See Tumor." From the term "Tumor" in the Alphabetic Index, the coder is directed to Back/Flank and Radical Resection. 21935.

3. After an injection of Lidocaine, the surgeon performed a percutaneous tenotomy (Achilles tendon). Refer to 27605–27606. What is the correct code assignment?

   Answer: Lidocaine is a local anesthesia; therefore, code 27605 is assigned.

4. Using cryosurgery, the surgeon removed four (4) dermatofibromas of the leg. Refer to CPT codes 17000–17250. What would be the correct code assignment?

   Answer: Dermatofibromas are benign. Code 17110 should be assigned.

5. Refer to codes 57550–57556. The surgeon performed an excision of a cervical stump, vaginally, with repair of an enterocele. What is the correct code assignment?

   Answer: 57556. The description for this code would be: *Excision of cervical stump, vaginal approach; with repair of enterocele.*

6. Insertion of a Foley catheter (temporary)

   Index: Insertion, Catheter, urethra
   (Foley is a type of urinary catheter.)

   Code: 51702

7. Biopsy of lacrimal sac

   Index: Biopsy, lacrimal sac

   Code: 68525

8. Incision and drainage, hematoma, sublingual, masticator space

   Index: Abscess, Mouth, Incision and drainage

   Code: 41018

Chapter 3
Modifiers

Matching Exercise

1. ____ 3P (C)   A. Physical status (anesthesia) modifier

2. ____ F4 (B)   B. HCPCS National modifier

3. ____ 73 (D)   C. Category II modifier

4. ____ P5 (A)   D. CPT Modifier Approved for Hospital Outpatient Use only

5. ____ 53 (E)   E. CPT Modifier not Approved for Hospital Outpatient Use

Select the Modifier Exercise

1. Patient is seen in the physician's office for his yearly physical (CPT code 99395–*Preventive Medicine E/M*). During the exam, the patient requests that the physician remove a mole on his shoulder. What CPT modifier would be appended to the 99395 to explain that the E/M service was unrelated to excision of the mole?

    Answer: Modifier 25

2. Patient is seen in a radiology clinic for an X-ray of the arm (73090). The films are sent to another radiologist (not affiliated with the clinic) to interpret and write the report. What HCPCS Level II modifier would be appended to the CPT code for the services of the radiology clinic?

    Answer: TC for Technical Component

3. A surgeon performed an esophageal dilation (43453) on a 4-week-old newborn who weighed 3.1 kg. What CPT modifier would be appended to CPT code to describe this special circumstance?

    Answer: 63 Procedure Performed on Infants less than 4 kg

4. The surgeon performed a tenolysis, extensor tendon of the right index finger (26445). What HCPCS Level II modifier should be appended to the CPT code?

    Answer: F6 Right hand, second digit

5. A planned arthroscopic meniscectomy of knee was planned for a patient. During the procedure, the scope was inserted but the patient went into respiratory distress and the procedure was terminated. What CPT modifier would be appended to the CPT code (29880) for the physician's services?

    Answer: 53 Discontinued Procedure. This modifier would be appended to the planned procedure for *physician services*.

Coding/Modifier Exercise

Case Study #1

The surgeon performed a carpal tunnel release (median nerve) on the left and right wrist.

> **Index: Carpal Tunnel syndrome**
>
> **Code: 64721–50 (modifier for bilateral)**

Case Study #2

A 45-year-old male is brought to the endoscopy suite for diagnostic EGD. Patient is prepped. After moving the patient to the procedure room, and prior to initiation of sedation, he develops significant hypotension, and the physician cancels the procedure. Code for hospital services.

> **Index: Endoscopy, Gastrointestinal, Upper, Exploration**
>
> **Code: 43235–73 Diagnostic EGD (modifier for Discontinued outpatient procedure prior to anesthesia administration)**

Case Study #3

The surgeon performed a tonsillectomy and adenoidectomy on a 25-year-old male. Four hours after leaving the surgery center, the patient presents to the clinic with a 1-hour history of bleeding in the throat. The bleeding site was located; however, it was in a location that could not be treated outside the OR. The patient was taken back to the OR for control of postoperative bleeding.

> **Index: Tonsillectomy and Hemorrhage, Throat**
>
> **Codes:**
> **42821 Tonsillectomy and adenoidectomy, age 12 years or older**
>
> **42962–78 Control oropharyngeal hemorrhage with secondary surgical intervention (Modifier for return to OR for a related procedure during the postoperative period)**

Case Study #4

> Patient presented for capsule endoscopy of the GI tract. The ileum was not visualized.
>
> **Index: Gastrointestinal Tract, Imaging, Intraluminal**
>
> **Code: 91110–52 GI tract imaging, intraluminal (Modifier for reduced services. The capsule endoscopy should include visualization from the esophagus through ileum.)**

Chapter 4
Surgery: Part I

Integumentary System Exercises

Medical Terminology Review

1. ____ biopsy (C)   A. freeze tissue
2. ____ basal cell carcinoma (D)   B. removal of damaged tissue from wound
3. ____ cryosurgery (A)   C. removal of a piece of tissue for examination
4. ____ debridement (B)   D. malignant neoplasm
5. ____ lipoma (E)   E. benign neoplasm

Case Studies

Case Study #1

With the use of a YAG laser, the surgeon removed a 2.0 cm Giant congenital melanocytic nevus of the leg. Pathology confirmed that the lesion was premalignant.

Index: Lesion, Skin, Destruction, Premalignant (Note that laser is classified as destruction and the morphology of the lesion is premalignant.)

Code: 17000 Destruction, premalignant; first lesion

Case Study #2

Operative Note: After local anesthesia was administered, the site was cleansed and an incision is made in the center of the sebaceous cyst. The cyst is drained and irrigated with a sterile solution. Diagnosis: sebaceous cyst of back.

Index: Incision and Drainage, Cyst, Skin

Code: 10060 Incision and drainage of abscess, cyst; simple

Case Study #3

Surgeon reports that the patient has a 2.0 cm basal cell carcinoma of the chin. The excision required removal of 0.5 cm margins around the lesion.

Index: Lesion, skin, excision, malignant.

Code: 11643 (size is 2.0 + .5 + .5 = 3.0 excised diameter)

Case Study #4

Physician performs a simple avulsion of the nail plate, second and third digits of the left foot.

Index: Nail, Avulsion

Codes: 11730–T1, 11732–T2 (11732 is an add-on code, used to identify additional nail plates.)

Case Study #5

Operative Procedure: Shaving of a 0.5 cm pyogenic granuloma of the neck

Index: Lesion, skin, shaving (Note that a pyogenic granuloma is a benign lesion; characterized as a red papule.)

Code: 11305 Shaving of dermal lesion, single

Case Study #6

Patient seen in the Emergency Department after an accident. A 3.0 cm wound of the upper arm required a layered closure and a 1.0 cm superficial laceration of the left cheek was repaired.

Index: Wound, Repair (Intermediate and Simple) Layered closures indicates an intermediate repair. Superficial indicates a simple repair.

Codes:
12032 Intermediate repair (extremities) 2.6 to 7.5 cm

12011 Simple repair, face, 2.5 cm or less

Case Study #7

Operative Note: Patient seeking treatment for a cyst of left breast. A 21-gauge needle was inserted into the cyst. The white, cystic fluid was aspirated and the needle withdrawn. Pressure was applied to the wound and the site covered with a bandage.

Index: Breast, Cyst, Puncture Aspiration

Code: 19000–LT Puncture aspiration of cyst of breast

Case Study #8

The surgeon fulgurates a .5 cm superficial basal cell carcinoma of the back.

Index: Lesion, Skin, Destruction, Malignant (Fulguration is a destruction technique; basal cell carcinoma is malignant.)

Code: 17260 Destruction, malignant lesion, trunk, 0.5 cm or less

Case Study #9

Operative Note: This 59-year-old male developed a sebaceous cyst on his right upper back. After ensuring a comfortable position, the skin surrounding the cyst was infiltrated with $\frac{1}{2}$% Xylocaine with epinephrine to achieve local anesthesia. An elliptical incision surrounding the cyst was made; total excised diameter of 5.0 cm. The cyst wall was dissected free from the surrounding tissues. Hemostatis was obtained and the wound was copiously irrigated. The wound was closed with 3-0 Vicryl, figure-of-eight stitches.

Abstract from Documentation:

What type of lesion was removed? Benign or malignant? **Sebaceous cyst—benign lesion (Upper back is listed as trunk in CPT.)**

How was it removed? **Excised**

What is the excised diameter of the lesion? **Size of lesion = 5.0 cm**

Did the physician close the wound routinely or was there a layered closure?
Note: Routine wound closure (included in CPT code), no mention of layered closure

Time to Code:

Index: Lesion, Skin, Excision, Benign (11400–11471)

Coding Assignment: 11406 (Excision, benign lesion, trunk, excised diameter over 4.0)

Case Study #10

Operative Report

Preoperative Diagnosis: 1.0 cm malignant melanoma, right heel

Postoperative Diagnosis: Same

Operation: Wide local excision with split thickness skin graft from the left thigh

Anesthesia: Spinal

Indications: This 72-year-old patient has a 1.0 cm malignant lesion of the left heel. He has agreed to a wide local excision.

Procedure: The patient was taken to the operating room, prepped and draped in the usual sterile fashion. A 1/20 of an inch thick split-thickness skin graft (7 cm $\times$ 7 cm) was harvested from the left thigh and preserved. Next, the lesion, which was on the medial aspect of the right heel, was excised with 2.5 cm margins down to and including some of the plantar fascia. Total excised diameter was 6.0 cm. Hemostatis was achieved with 2-0 Tycron sutures and the cautery. After suitable hemostasis was obtained, the wound margins were advanced with interrupted sutures of 2-0 chromic and then the skin graft was placed.

The skin graft was approximated to the skin using interrupted running sutures of 4-0 chromic, and then holes were punched in the skin graft to permit egress of serous fluid. Then, a bolster dressing of cotton batting wrapped in Owen's gauze was placed over the skin graft site and secured to the skin with multiple sutures tied over it to 2-0 Tycron. The skin graft donor site was wrapped with Owen's gauze, two moistened ABD pads and wrapped with a Kerlix and an Ace wrap. The patient tolerated the procedure well and was transported awake and alert to the recovery room in excellent condition

Abstract from Documentation:

What procedure was performed? Excision of lesion and skin graft to cover the defect

What are the excised diameter, location and type (malignant/benign) of lesion: Malignant lesion of left heel—lesion was 1.0 c, but 2.5 cm margins were obtained (1.0 + 2.5 + 2.5 = 6.0 cm lesion).

What is the coding guideline that for coding excision of lesion with subsequent skin replacement surgery? Do you code both or just the skin graft? When an excision of a lesion requires a skin replacement/substitute graft for repair of the defect, the coder should assign the excision of lesion code in addition to the graft.

What type of skin graft was performed? Adjacent? Skin Replacement? Autograft? Cultured tissue? Free (autologous) from thigh to cover defect of heel

Was the skin graft full-thickness or split-thickness? Split-thickness.

For coding purposes, identify site of defect, size and type of graft: Split-thickness, autograft, heel and less than 100 sq cm (size of skin removed was 7 × 7 cm)

Time to Code:

Index for Excision of Lesion: Lesion, Skin, Excision, Malignant

Index for Skin Graft: Skin, Graft, Free

Code Assignment:
15120 Split-thickness autograft, feet, first 100 sq. cm or less

11626 Excision, malignant lesion, feet, over 4.0 cm

Musculoskeletal System Exercises

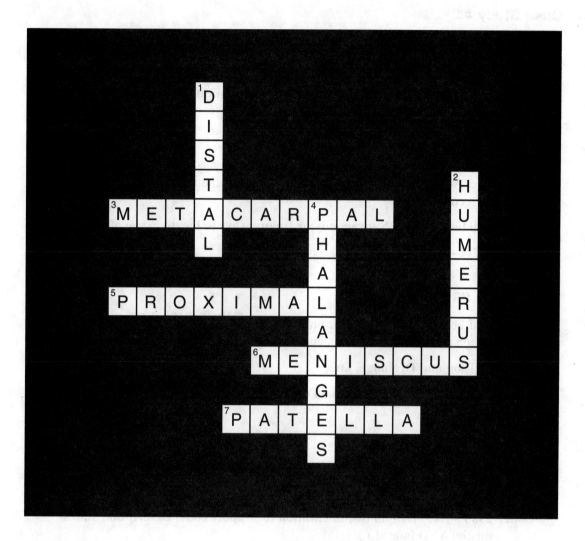

Across

3. Bones of hand [METACARPAL]
5. Near center of body [PROXIMAL]
6. Cartilage in knee joint [MENISCUS]
7. Knee bone [PATELLA]

Down

1. Away from center of body [DISTAL]
2. Bone of upper arm [HUMERUS]
4. Bones of fingers or toes [PHALANGES]

Case Studies

Case Study #1

The surgeon performed a closed reduction of a scapular fracture.

> **Index: Fracture, scapula, closed treatment, with manipulation**

> **Code: 23575 (Note that reduction indicates that manipulation was performed.)**

Case Study #2

The patient is seen in the outpatient surgery department for a comminuted left supracondylar femoral fracture. An open reduction and internal fixation of the left supracondylar femur fracture was performed.

> **Index: Fracture, Femur, Supracondylar (many ways to locate range of Codes)**

> **Code: 27511–LT**

Case Study #3

The patient had been diagnosed with an infected abscess extending below the fascia of the knee. The surgeon performed an incision and drainage of the abscess.

> **Index: Incision and Drainage, knee**

> **Code: 27301 (Deep abscess based on documentation of below the fascia.)**

Case Study #4

The surgeon performed an arthroscopy of the right knee with medial and lateral meniscectomy.

> **Index: Arthroscopy, surgical, knee**

> **Code: 29880–RT (Need all documentation to support code. Description states medial AND lateral.)**

Case Study #5

The surgeon performed a percutaneous tenotomy of the left hand, second digit and third digit.

> **Index: Tenotomy, finger**

> **Codes: 26060–F1 and 26060–F2**

Case Study #6

Surgeon performed an arthroscopy of the right knee with limited synovectomy and shaving of articular cartilage.

> **Index: Arthroscopy, surgical, knee**

> **Code: 29877–RT (Code 29875 should not be assigned. It is a "separate procedure," integral part of procedure.)**

Case Study #7

A patient is diagnosed with osteochondroma of the scapula. The surgeon excises the tumor.

Abstract from Documentation:

What is an osteochondroma? **Benign bone tumor**

Time to Code:

Index: Tumor, Scapula, Excision (Osteochondroma is benign.)

Code: 23140

Case Study #8

Emergency Department Report

Chief Complaint: Left wrist injury

History of Present Illness: The patient is a 5-year-old female who presents in the ED after accidentally falling off her bicycle. She tried to brace her fall with her left wrist and now says there is pain that increases with movement. She had no other injuries. There were no head injuries.

Vital Signs: Blood pressure 117/72, temperature 97.8, pulse 106, respirations 20

General: The patient is alert, oriented × 3 in no acute distress seated in the hospital bed.

Extremities: Physical exam of the left upper extremity reveals no deformity. To palpation the patient has tenderness of the distal radius and ulna. No tenderness to palpation of the hand. Range of motion is limited in the wrist but intact in the hand and elbow with no tenderness in the elbow.

Emergency Room Course: X-ray of the left wrist revealed a Buckle fracture of the distal radius and ulna. Volar splint and sling were applied. The patient was discharged.

Assessment: Buckle fracture left distal radius and ulna

Plan: Ice and elevate, return if worse, follow-up with orthopedics in 2–3 days, Tylenol with codeine elixir p.r.n. for pain was prescribed.

Abstract from Documentation:

What was the treatment for the fracture? **Applied Volar splint**

Time to Code:

Index: Splint, arm, short

Code: 29125–LT Application of short arm splint (forearm to hand) static (Note that static is used for immobilization of the injury; dynamic allows for mobilization.)

Case Study #9

Operative Report

Preoperative Diagnosis: Right arm mass

Postoperative Diagnosis: Right arm mass

Procedure: Excision, right arm mass

Indications: This is a 42-year-old woman who presents with palpable enlarging uncomfortable mass in the right upper arm. After discussion, she agreed with excision of the area.

Anesthesia: Local with 1% plain Lidocaine and sedation

Blood Loss: Minimal

Details of Procedure: After informed consent was obtained, the patient was taken to the operating room and placed on the table in supine position. Sedation was administered and the right arm was prepped with Betadine solution and draped sterilely. The palpable mass was identified and an elliptical skin incision was created over the mass along its axis and the underlying mass was excised in its entirety to the level of muscle fascia. It appeared to be most consistent with being multi-lobulated lipoma. It was forwarded to Pathology. The wound was inspected for hemostasis, which was excellent. The deep tissues were approximated with interrupted 3-0 Vicryl and running 4-0 Monocryl subcuticular stitch was used to approximate the skin edges. Benzoin, Steri-Strips and sterile dressing were applied. She was awakened from sedation and returned to the recovery room in stable condition having tolerated the procedure well.

Pathology Report

Final Diagnosis: Soft tissue mass of right upper arm. Lipoma

Gross Description: Received in formalin labeled "lipoma of right arm" consists of a 7 × 4 × 2.5 cm yellow lobulated encapsulated portion of adipose tissue with an overlying 4 × 1.5 cm strip of tan heavily wrinkled unremarkable skin.

Abstract from Documentation:

What was the final diagnosis from the pathologist? **Lipoma—right upper arm**

How deep did the mass extend? **Into muscle fascia**

What was the treatment for the mass? **Excision**

Is this a removal of a skin tumor or did it extend into the musculoskeletal area? **Deep in the fascia—beyond the skin**

Time to Code:

Index: Tumor, Arm, Upper, Excision (-oma means tumor)

Code: 24076–RT

Case Study #10

Operative Report

Preoperative Diagnosis: Mechanical complication from internal 0.062 K wire, first metatarsal, right foot

Postoperative Diagnosis: Same

Procedure: Removal of K wire, right foot

The patient was brought to the operating room and placed on the table in supine position under the influence of IV sedation. The local anesthesia was administered. The right foot was prepped and draped in the usual sterile fashion. The right foot was exsanguinated with an Esmarch bandage and his ankle tourniquet was inflated. A 1 cm dorsal medial skin incision was made directly over the palpable head of the pin. The incision was deepened bluntly, taking care to preserve and retract neurovascular structures. The periosteum was sharply incised from the underlying pin, and the pin was removed with a large straight hemostat. The wound was flushed with copious amounts of sterile normal saline. The skin was reapproximated with a 5-0 Vicryl in a subcuticular fashion. The site was dressed with Xeroform gauze and a dry sterile compression dressing. 4 cc of 0.5% Marcaine was injected for postoperative anesthesia.

Abstract from Documentation:

What is a K wire? **Pin fixation to hold bone fragments together.**

What procedure was performed for this patient? **Removal of pin**

Time to Code:

Index: Removal, fixation device

Code: 20680–RT Removal of implant; deep (buried pin)

Respiratory System Exercises

Medical Terminology Review

1. ____ larynx (E)   A. major air passages of lungs

2. ____ esophagus (C)   B. connects mouth to esophagus

3. ____ bronchus (A)   C. structure leads from throat to stomach

4. ____ pharynx (B)   D. a bone in the nose

5. ____ ethmoid (D)   E. voicebox

Case Studies

Case Study #1

The surgeon performed a thoracoscopy for a wedge resection of the lung.

Index: Thoracoscopy, Surgical, with Wedge Resection of lung

Code: 32657

Case Study #2

Bronchoscopy with multiple transbronchial lung biopsies taken of the right upper lobe.

Index: Bronchoscopy, biopsy

Code: 31628 Bronchoscopy with transbronchial lung biopsy(s), single lobe (Although several biopsies were performed they were of the small lobe.)

Case Study #3

Patient seen in the Emergency Department for epistaxis. Physician performs an anterior packing of left nasal passage.

Index: Epistaxis

Code: 30901–LT Control nasal hemorrhage, anterior, simple

Case Study #4

Physician performs a bilateral nasal endoscopy with total ethmoidectomy.

Index: Endoscopy, Nose, Surgical

Code: 31255–50

Case Study #5

Patient is seen with difficulty breathing due to deviated nasal septum. The surgeon performs a submucous resection of the septum.

> **Index: Nasal Septum, Submucous Resection (Resection directs coder to see Nasal Septum.)**

> **Code: 30520**

Case Study #6

The surgeon performs a thoracentesis by placing a needle through the chest wall into pleura to withdraw fluid, which will be sent to the lab for analysis.

> **Index: Thoracentesis (provides a range of codes)**

> **Code: 32421 Thoracentesis, puncture of pleural cavity for aspiration, initial or subsequent**

Case Study #7

A patient was diagnosed with squamous cell carcinoma of the larynx. The surgeon performed a supraglottic laryngectomy with radical neck dissection to remove the metastasis to the lymph nodes.

> **Index: Laryngectomy (Supraglottic procedure preserves part of the voice box.)**

> **Code: 31368 Laryngectomy; subtotal supraglottic, with radical neck dissection**

Case Study #8

Operative Report

Preoperative Diagnosis: Chronic laryngitis with polypoid disease

Postoperative Diagnosis: Same

Procedure: Direct laryngoscopy and removal of polyps from both cords

Procedure Detail: After adequate premedication, the patient was taken to the operating room and placed in supine position. The Jako laryngoscope was inserted. There were noted to be large polyps on both vocal cords, essentially obstructing the glottic airway. Using the straight-cup forceps, the polyps were removed from the left cord first. They were removed up to the anterior third, but the anterior tip was not removed on the left side. The polyps were removed from the right cord up to the anterior commissure. There was minimal bleeding noted. The patient was extubated and sent to recovery in good condition.

Abstract from Documentation:

> *What type of endoscopy was performed?* **Laryngoscopy—direct**

> *What procedure was performed during the endoscopy?* **Removal of polyps**

Time to Code:

> **Index: Laryngoscopy, endoscopy, excision**

> **Code: 31540 Laryngoscopy, direct, operative with excision of tumor**

Case Study #9

Operative Report

Preoperative Diagnosis: Abnormal chest X-ray and CT scan revealed possible malignant neoplasm of the right upper lobe. Patient is a heavy smoker.

Postoperative Diagnosis: Squamous cell carcinoma, upper right lobe

Procedure: Flexible Bronchoscopy

Procedure: The patient was prepped, draped and after adequate anesthesia, the scope was inserted through the right nares. The scope was advanced further. The vocal cords were normal. Carina was normal. The right main bronchus up into the upper middle and lower lobe bronchi were visualized. The right upper lobe showed an obstructive lesion. Other segments of the middle and lower lobe bronchi were normal. Biopsies and brushings were taken from the right upper lobe bronchus. The patient tolerated the procedure well.

Abstract from Documentation:

What procedures were performed during the endoscopic procedure? **Biopsies and brushing**

Time to Code:

Index: Bronchoscopy, Biopsy & Bronchoscopy, brushings

Codes:
31625 Bronchoscopy with bronchial biopsy(s)

31623 With brushings

(Note: in a physician setting, modifier 51 would be appended to the 31623 code.)

Case Study #10

Operative Report

Preoperative Diagnosis: Bilateral true vocal cord lesions

Postoperative Diagnosis: Bilateral true vocal cord intracordal cyst

Operation: Microlaryngoscopy and biopsy

Indications: This is a 58-year-old man with a history of tobacco use who has had a hoarse voice for the past couple of years. The patient also has an alcohol history. Considering his risk factors and hoarseness, the patient agreed to undergo the surgical procedure to not only better define the lesion but also the nature of the lesion by getting biopsies for pathology.

Operative Findings: Bilateral intracordal mucoid cysts without any evidence of ulcerations or other mass lesions of the vocal cords

Details of Procedure: Patient was brought to the operating room and laid supine on the operating table. After adequate anesthesia, a Dedo laryngoscope was used to survey the supraglottic area. Once other abnormalities were ruled out, attention was then directed to the true vocal cords. The patient was then suspended using the Dedo laryngoscope and the operating microscope was then brought into the field. Under binocular microscopy the nature of the lesions were better assessed. It appeared that the vocal cords themselves were smooth and very soft to palpation. A boucher retractor was then used to grasp the right true vocal cord and a sickle knife was then used to make an incision laterally. Left-going scissors were then used to create a submucosal flap. The mucoid mass was then extruded and grasped with the non-traumatic graspers and the scissors were then used to dissect the full extent of the mass. The suction was then used to verify the operative site on the right true vocal cord, and once adequate resection was achieved, the mucosal flap was then placed back onto normal position. Attention was then given towards the left intracordal cyst, which was not as prominent as the right. Again using left nontraumatic graspers the left true vocal cord was grasped and medialized with enough tension so that the sickle knife could be used to make an incision laterally. A submucosal flap was then developed using the suction tip and the mucosal cyst was then identified and carefully excised from the tissues of the true vocal cord, careful not to violate the ligaments or get into the vocals muscle. At this point, once adequate excision was obtained, the mucosal flap was then replaced. At this time, Afrin-soaked pledgets were then used to create adequate hemostasis. The Afrin-soaked pledgets were then removed at the conclusion of the operation. The operating microscope was then taken out the field. The patient was then taken out of suspension and his care was then handed over to the anesthesiologist.

Abstract from Documentation:

What type of endoscopy was performed? **Laryngoscopy**

What was performed during the endoscopic procedure? **Excision of mucoid mass and excision of cyst (for CPT coding purposes, these are refer to as "tumors"—generic term for growths).**

Time to Code:

Index: Laryngoscopy, Operative

Code: 31541 Laryngoscopy, direct, operative with operating microscope (only coded once even though more than one cyst was removed. Note the physician used an operating microscope.)

Cardiovascular System Exercises

Medical Terminology Review

1. ____ fistula (C)   A. surgically closing off a vessel
2. ____ graft (D)   B. blood clot
3. ____ stenosis (E)   C. surgically made passage
4. ____ thrombus (B)   D. piece of tissue that is transplanted surgically
5. ____ ligation (A)   E. narrowing of a passage

Case Studies

Case Study #1

Surgeon performed a quadruple coronary artery bypass using a saphenous vein.

> **Index: Coronary Artery Bypass (range)**
>
> **Code: 33513 Coronary artery bypass, vein only; four coronary venous grafts**

Case Study #2

Operative Note

Diagnosis: End-stage renal disease

Procedure: Creation of left forearm arterial venous fistula

The patient was prepped and draped in the usual manner. An incision was made over the radial artery and cephalic vein. Each was dissected free to create an anastomosis.

> **Index: Anastomosis, Arteriovenous Fistula, Direct** *(Difficult to find in the index if you search under creation or AV fistula.)*
>
> **Code: 36821–LT Arteriovenous anastomosis, open; direct, any site** *(The professional edition of CPT has a illustration of this procedure.)*

Case Study #3

Operative Note

Diagnosis: Thrombosis of right AV (Gore-Tex) graft

Procedure: A transverse incision was made in order to complete a thrombectomy of the graft. Because the balloon catheter could not be passed, it was elected to perform an arteriotomy for removal of the thrombus. The area was irrigated and the incision was closed.

> Index: Thrombectomy, Arteriovenous Fistula, Graft leads to a percutaneous thrombectomy code. This is an open approach since the arteriotomy was performed. See in index: Thrombectomy, Dialysis Graft, without Revision.
>
> Code: 36831 Thrombectomy, open, arteriovenous fistula without revision, autogenous or nonautogenous dialysis graft

Case Study #4

A patient with a previously implanted pacing cardioverter-defibrillator now requires repositioning of the device.

> Index: Repositioning, Heart, Defibrillator, Leads
>
> Code: 33215 Repositioning of previously implanted transvenous pacemaker or pacing cardioverter-defibrillator

Case Study #5

Surgeon performs a percutaneous transluminal angioplasty on the femoral-popliteal artery for a patient with coronary artery disease.

> Index: Percutaneous Transluminal Angioplasty, Artery, Femoral-Popliteal
>
> Code: 35474

Case Study #6

Surgeon performs an axillary-brachial thromboendarterectomy with patch graft.

> Index: Thromboendarterectomy, Axillary Artery
>
> Code: 35321

Case Study #7

Operative Note

Procedure: Permanent pacemaker implantation

Details of Procedure: The patient was prepped and draped in the usual sterile fashion. The left subclavian vein was accessed, and the guidewire was placed in position. A deep subcutaneous pacemaker pocket was created using the blunt dissection technique. A French 7 introducer sheath was advanced over the guidewire, and the guidewire was removed. A bipolar endocardial lead model was advanced under fluoroscopic guidance and tip of pacemaker lead was positioned in the right ventricular apex.

Next, the French-9.5 introducer sheath was advanced over a separate guidewire under fluoroscopic guidance, and guide wire was removed.

Through this sheath, a bipolar atrial screw-in lead was positioned in the right atrial appendage, and the lead was screwed in.

Abstract from Documentation:

What is the coding selection for a permanent pacemaker? **Review of the index reveals the selection as 33206–33207.**

What documentation determines the correct code selection? **If insertion is in the atrium, ventricle or both. In this case it is both.**

Time to Code:

Index: Insertion, Pacemaker Heart

Codes: 33208 Insertion, atrial and ventricular

Case Study #8

With an incision into the arm, the surgeon repaired a ruptured false aneurysm of axillary-brachial artery.

Index: Aneurysm Repair, Brachial Artery

Code: 35013 Direct repair for ruptured aneurysm, axillary-brachial artery, by arm incision

Case Study #9

Operative Report

Preoperative Diagnosis: Severe left common iliac artery stenosis with claudication

Postoperative Diagnosis: Same

Procedure: Angioplasty of left common iliac artery stenosis

Through a left groin, a 7 French Cordis introducer was placed after the lesion had been crossed with the guidewire. A 9 mm × 4 cm balloon was then chosen. The patient was given 2,000 units of heparin intra-arterially. The balloon was then positioned in the proper location and gently inflated. The stenosis dilated easily. The balloon was inflated for one minute and then brought down. The catheter was advanced, the guidewire removed, and completion angiography revealed satisfactory dilatation with no stenosis. The patient was taken to the recovery room in satisfactory condition.

Abstract from Documentation:

What main procedure was performed? **Repair of stenosis**

What was technique was used to eliminate the stenosis? **Balloon angioplasty**

Time to Code:

Index: Angioplasty, Iliac Artery, Percutaneous (*no incision, guidewire used to percutaneously insert the balloon*)

Code: 35473

Case Study #10

Preoperative Diagnosis: Status post Port-a-Cath

Postoperative Diagnosis: Same

Procedure: Removal of Port-a-Cath

Indications: The patient has completed the chemotherapy treatment and elects to remove the Port-a-Cath.

Procedure: The patient was placed in supine position. Right subclavian area was prepped and adequately draped. Local anesthesia was given just over the port, transverse incision was made. Skin incision was deepened down to port area. Fibrinous capsule was exposed and retracted and sharply dissected to remove the soft tissue. Entire fibrinous capsule was excised and then the tunnel was clamped and tied off from the fibrinous capsule, after the entire system was removed. The area was irrigated. Hemostasis was assured. Subcutaneous layer was closed using 4-0. Skin was approximated using 5-0 Vicryl running stitches. Steri-strips applied. Patient tolerated the procedure well.

Abstract from Documentation:

Review CPT Notes preceding the coding section for central venous access procedures.

What is a port-a-cath? Venous access device

What was the operative action? The port was removed.

Time to Code:

Index: Removal, Venous Access Device

Code: 36590 Removal of tunneled central venous access device with subcutaneous port

Digestive System Exercises

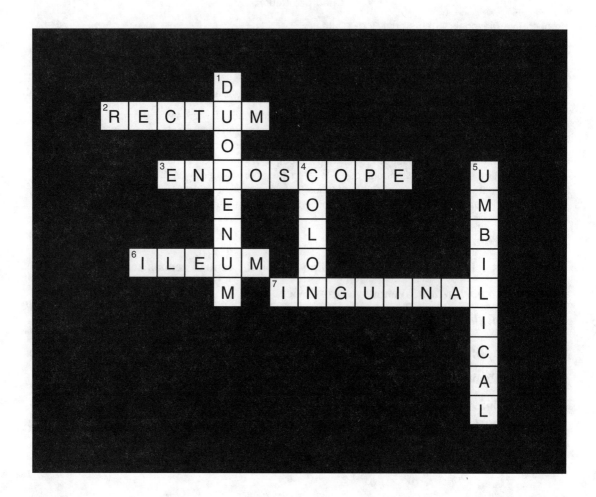

Across

2. Final section of large intestine [RECTUM]
3. Instrument to view inside body [ENDOSCOPE]
6. Third portion of small intestines [ILEUM]
7. Groin [INGUINAL]

Down

1. First part of small intestine [DUODENUM]
4. From cecum to rectum [COLON]
5. Navel [UMBILICAL]

Case Studies

Case Study #1

Operative Report

Preoperative Diagnosis: Inadequate p.o. intake.

Postoperative Diagnosis: Same

Operation: Percutaneous endoscopic gastrostomy tube placement.

Anesthesia: IV sedation

Clinical History: The patient is a 75-year-old female patient with inadequate p.o. intake who presents now for PEG tube placement.

Operative Procedure: After establishment of an adequate level of IV sedation and viscous spray of the oropharynx, EGD scope was inserted without difficulty to the second portion of the duodenum from whence it was gradually withdrawn. There were no striking duodenal findings. The pylorus appeared unremarkable and on visualization, the antrum, body and fundus of the stomach were also unremarkable. With withdrawal of the scope, the esophagus and GE junction visualized normal. Insufflation of the stomach was undertaken and at point of maximal transillumination in the epigastrium, local infiltration was undertaken by Dr. June and a slit incision was made. Needle within a cannula was then threaded percutaneously directly into the stomach under visualization. Inner cannula was removed and guidewire was passed. Loop forceps were then passed endoscopically, and guidewire was grasped in the stomach and brought out orally, whence it was anchored to a PEG tube which was pulled to emanate via the anterior abdominal wall being anchored to appropriate position.

The patient tolerated the procedure well. There were no complications.

> **Index: Gastrostomy Tube, Placement, Percutaneous Endoscopic**
>
> **Code: 43246**

Case Study #2

Operative Note: The patient is morbidly obese with a BMI of 37. Procedure performed: Laparoscopic insertion of gastric band.

> **Index: Laparoscopy, Gastric Restrictive Procedures**
>
> **Code: 43770**

Case Study #3

Diagnosis: Esophageal stricture

Procedure: Upper endoscopy with esophageal dilation

Indications for Procedure: The patient is a 65-year-old woman who has a known esophageal stricture that has required periodic dilation in the past. She has recently had recurrent difficulty with solid food.

Operative Procedure: The instrument was passed easily into the esophagus. The esophagus had normal mucosa. The gastroesophageal junction was present at 30 cm where there was a stricture present and extended for no more than a couple of millimeters in length.

There was a single linear erosion extending about 1 cm above, consistent with reflux esophagitis. Below the stricture, there was a 4-cm sliding hiatal hernia. On retroversion, no additional abnormalities were noted. The body of the stomach distended well and had a normal rugal pattern. The antrum was briefly seen and was normal, as were the duodenal bulb and descending duodenum.

The instrument was withdrawn into the stomach, and a Savary guidewire was passed under direct vision with fluoroscopic control. The instrument was withdrawn, and the patient was dilated with the passage of the 15-, 17-, and 20-mm Savary dilators with minimal resistance encountered and no heme on the dilators.

Abstract from Documentation:

What exactly was visualized during this endoscopic procedure? **Esophagus, stomach and duodenum (EGD)**

Besides visualization (diagnostic endoscopy) what else was performed during the endoscopy)? **Nothing. The dilation occurred after the scope was withdrawn.**

Time to Code:

Index:

> **1. Endoscopy, Gastrointestinal, Upper, Exploration**
>
> **2. Dilation, Esophagus**

Codes:

> **43235 (EGD)**
>
> **43450–59 Dilation of esophagus**

Case Study #4

Operative Report

Operation: Ventral hernia repair with mesh Marlex

History: This is a 45-year-old white male who came in complaining of a bulging mass in the right side of the abdomen. He is a surgical candidate for an initial hernia repair.

Operative Technique: Under general anesthesia, the patient was prepped and draped in the usual fashion. A midline incision from the xiphoid to the suprapubic area was carried out. A lateral flap was developed on the right side as well as the left side. The umbilicus was isolated with an elliptical incision. After completion of the flap and identification of the fascia, there was found a big gap in the midline as well as in the right side of the abdomen. At this point, we proceeded to perform plication of the rectus abdominis muscle. Subsequent to that, we applied the mesh Marlex around the area. Next, we left two Jackson-Pratt drains in the subcutaneous tissue. The redundant skin was resected, and the umbilicus was closed in this area. To close the abdominal wall, we used staples, and for the periumbilical area we used interrupted nylon 3-0. Bleeding was minimal. Condition was good. The patient tolerated the procedure very well and left the operating room in good and stable condition.

Abstract from Documentation:

What is a ventral hernia? **Also known as incisional. An incisional hernia occurs in the abdomen in the area of an old surgical scar.**

What are the coding guidelines for assigning the implantation of mesh code with a hernia repair? **It is only assigned for use with incisional or ventral hernia repair. It would be applicable in this case.**

Time to Code:

Index:

1. **Hernia Repair** *(Note that the CPT index does not have an entry for Ventral. Incisional is another name for ventral, but the index is lacking in a general entry for incisional hernia. The choices are Incisional, Incarcerated (incorrect) or Recurrent Incisional (incorrect). Best to reference Hernia, Abdomen, Incisional.)*

2. **Mesh, Implantation, Hernia**

Codes:

49560 Repair initial incisional or ventral hernia, reducible

49568 Implantation of mesh

Case Study #5

Emergency Department Record

Chief Complaint: Foreign body in throat

History of Present Illness: This is a 73-year-old male who has a history of esophageal stricture, who has had multiple endoscopies to have foreign bodies removed. He was eating roast beef last night and it stuck in his throat. He says anything he tries to eat or drink comes right back up. He called Dr. Ida early this morning and stated that he would meet him in the emergency room. Patient denies any chest pain, fever, chills, shortness of breath or other systemic complaints.

Dr. Ida did an endoscopy and removed several pieces of meat as well as a pea. The patient did receive conscious sedation for the procedure. We watched him in the emergency room on his recovery.

Impressions: Meat impaction in esophagus.

Index: Endoscopy, esophagus, Removal, Foreign Body

Code: 43215

Case Study #6

Operative Note

Procedure: Colonoscopy with biopsy

Indications: This 26-year-old female was referred for evaluation because of abdominal pain with occasional episodes of rectal bleeding and some mucus in the stool.

Procedure: The scope was inserted and advanced to the cecum. The rectum showed small pinpoint ulcers but nothing beyond that. I did take some biopsies. The sigmoid colon, descending, transverse and ascending colon was normal.

Index: Colonoscopy, Biopsy

Code: 45380 Colonoscopy with biopsies

Case Study #7

Operative Report

Preoperative Diagnosis: Thrombosed hemorrhoids

Postoperative Diagnosis: Same

Indications: This 25-year-old female, one week postpartum, complains of extremely painful hemorrhoids. Examination revealed circumferential prolapsed hemorrhoids with partial thrombosis in multiple areas.

Procedure: After induction of general anesthesia, she was prepped and draped in the usual sterile fashion. The patient was placed in lithotomy position and a retractor was placed in the anus. Very prominent, large, partially thrombosed external hemorrhoid was identified at 7-8 o'clock in the lithotomy position. It was grasped with a hemorrhoidal clamp. A 2-0 chromic stitch was placed at the apex. The Bovie electrocautery was then used to elliptically excise the large hemorrhoid, staying superficial to the sphincter muscle. Bleeding was controlled with Bovie electrocautery. The mucosa was closed with a running chromic stitch, leaving the end-point epidermis open.

Two other very large external hemorrhoids with thrombosis were then identified, at the 5 o'clock position in lithotomy and at the 10-11 o'clock position. These two hemorrhoids were excised in the exact same fashion as the first hemorrhoid. At the conclusion, there was no evidence of bleeding. The patient was returned to the recovery area in good condition.

Abstract from Documentation:

What method was used to remove the hemorrhoids? **Electrocautery (a form of destruction)**

Where the hemorrhoids internal or external? **External**

Time to Code:

Index: Hemorrhoid, Destruction

Code: 46935 Destruction of hemorrhoids, any method; external

Case Study #8

Operative Report

Procedure: Colonoscopy

Indications: Polyp seen on flexible sigmoidoscopy.

Procedure: After obtaining consent, the scope as passed under direct vision. Throughout the procedure, the patient's blood pressure, pulse, and oxygen saturations were monitored continuously. The Olympus pediatric colonoscopy was introduced through the anus and advanced to the ileum. The colonoscopy was accomplished without difficulty. The patient tolerated the procedure well

Findings: The terminal ileum was normal. Multiple small-mouthed diverticula were found in the sigmoid colon. A pedunculated polyp was found in the sigmoid colon. The polyp was 30 mm in size. Polypectomy was performed with hot snare after injecting 4cc of epinephrine in the stalk for hemostasis. Resection and retrieval were complete. Estimated blood loss was minimal.

Internal, non-bleeding, mild hemorrhoids were found.

Abstract from Documentation:

What this a diagnostic or surgical colonoscopy? **Surgical**

What technique was used to remove the polyp? **Hot snare**

Time to Code:

Index: Colonoscopy, Removal Tumor

Code: 45385 Colonoscopy with removal by snare technique

Case Study #9

Operative Report

Preoperative Diagnosis: Right colon cancer; probable liver metastasis

Postoperative Diagnosis: Cecal cancer, extensive bilateral liver metastasis

Procedures Performed: Right colectomy and biopsy of right lobe liver nodule

Indications: Patient is a 67-year-old man who presented with anemia. Colonoscopy demonstrated bleeding cecal carcinoma. CT scan suggested liver metastasis. He presents now for a palliative right colectomy and biopsy of liver nodule.

Description: The patient was brought to the operating room and placed in a supine position. Satisfactory general endotracheal anesthesia was achieved. He was prepped and draped exposing the anterior abdomen and a lower midline incision was created sharply through subcutaneous tissues by electrocautery. Linea alba was parted and exploration was performed. The right colon was mobilized by dissection in the avascular plane. The patient had three to four centimeter cecal cancer. The right ureter was identified and preserved.

The terminal ileum and distal ascending colon were divided with GIA-60 stapling devices. The right colic artery and lymph node tissue were resected back to the origin of the superior mesenteric artery with clamps and 3-0 silk ties. The specimen was forwarded to pathology. A stapled functional end-to-end anastomosis was then performed. The antimesenteric edges were reapproximated with a single fire of GIA-60 stapler. The defect created by the stapler was then closed with interrupted 3-0 silk Lembert sutures. The mesocolon was reapproximated with some interrupted 3-0 silk sutures. Hemostasis was confirmed. The right anterior liver nodule was biopsied with a Tru-Cut needle. Hemostasis was achieved. The midline fascia was closed with running 1-0 Prolene suture. The skin was approximated with staples. The wound was dressed. The procedure was concluded. The patient tolerated the procedure well and was taken to recovery in stable condition. Estimated blood loss was less than 100 cc. There were no complications.

Pathology Report

#1: Right Hemicolectomy: Adenocarcinoma of cecum

#2: Liver Biopsies: metastatic adenocarcinoma

Abstract from Documentation:

Locate the code selection for colectomy. What additional information is needed from the operative report to assign a correct code? **Partial or Total and additional procedures**

In the index, what code selection is provided for the liver biopsy? **47000, 47001, 47100**

What differentiates between these codes? **Percutaneous, performed at time of major procedure and if wedge biopsy was performed.**

Time to Code:

Index:

1. Colectomy, Partial with Anastomosis

2. Biopsy, Liver

Codes:

44140 Colectomy, partial; with anastomosis

47001 Biopsy of liver, needle; when done for indicated purpose at time of other major procedure (List separately in addition to code for primary procedure.)

Case Study #10

Operative Note

Diagnosis: Gallstone pancreatitis and biliary tree obstruction

Procedure: ERCP

Indications: The patient has gallstone pancreatitis, and an ultrasound showed a dilated common duct with stones.

Procedure: An ERCP with sphincterotomy was performed.

Index: ERCP send coders to See Bile Duct, Cholangiopancreatography; Pancreatic Duct, Bile Duct, Endoscopy, Incision, Sphincter

Code: 43262 ERCP; with sphincterotomy

Chapter 4
Surgery: Part II

Urinary System Exercises

Medical Terminology Review

1. ____ -lith (D)   A. sac that stores urine

2. ____ ureter (C)   B. duct leads urine out of body from bladder

3. ____ bladder (A)   C. duct from kidney to bladder

4. ____ kidney (E)   D. stone

5. ____ urethra (B)   E. organ that purifies blood and excretes waste in urine

Case Studies

Case Study #1

Using calibrated electronic equipment, an uroflowmetry test is performed to measure how well the bladder empties and the storage capacity of the bladder.

Index: Uroflowmetry

Code: 51741 Complex uroflowmetry

Case Study #2

Operative Note: Cystoscopy to remove stones from the patient's upper right ureter and another stone lodged in the middle left ureter. Both stones were manipulated back into the kidney with subsequent placement of double J ureteral stents in each ureter.

Index:
Cystourethroscopy, Manipulation of Ureteral Calculus

Cystourethroscopy, Insertion, Indwelling Ureteral Stent

(Note that Gibbons or double J are types of indwelling stents.)

Codes:
52330–50 Cystourethroscopy (including ureteral catheterization); with manipulation, without removal of ureteral calculus

52332–50 Cystourethroscopy, with insertion of indwelling ureteral stent *(Note that modifier 51 would be applicable for physician services.)*

Case Study #3

Operative Note: Patient has a ureteral stricture. Performed a cysto, ureteroscopy and laser treatment of the stricture.

Index: Cystourethroscopy, Dilation, Ureter

Code: 52344 Cystourethroscopy with ureteroscopy; with treatment of ureteral stricture

Case Study #4

Operative Note: Performed a cystoscopy with resection of a 2.0 cm bladder tumor. The procedure concluded with a steroid injection into the urethral stricture.

Index:
Bladder, Endoscopy, Excision, Tumor (results in code 52235)

Cystourethroscopy, with Steroid Injection

Codes
52235 Cystourethroscopy with fulguration and/or resection of medium bladder tumor (2.0 to 5.0 cm)

52283 Cystourethroscopy with steroid injection into stricture

(Note that modifier 51 would be appended to 52283 for physician services.)

Case Study #5

Operative Report

Preoperative Diagnosis: History of low grade transitional cell carcinoma

Postoperative Diagnosis: Same

Procedure: Flexible cystoscopy

Indications: Patient is a 49-year-old male diagnosed with low-grade transitional cell carcinoma of the bladder. He is here today for his regular bladder tumor follow-up.

Details: Patient's genitalia were prepped and draped in the typical fashion. 20 cc of 2% lidocaine jelly was instilled into the urethra. The anesthesia was given five minutes to set in. The #19 French flexible cystoscope was passed through the urethra into the bladder. Once inside the bladder, the entire bladder mucosa was evaluated. No lesions were identified. Both ureteral orifices were seen and were found to be normal. At this point, the scope was removed. Patient will be called in three months for his next follow-up.

Index: Cystourethroscopy

Code: 52000 Cystourethroscopy (separate procedure)

Case Study #6

Operative Report

Preoperative Diagnosis: Multiple bladder stones

Procedure: Cystoscopy with cystolitholapaxy

Indications: This 58-year-old patient was found to have several bladder stones. He is here today for removal of those stones. The patient is voiding well currently. Informed consent was signed and risks and benefits were explained, understood by the patient prior to the procedure. He agreed to proceed.

Description of Procedure: The patient was taken to the cystoscopy suite, placed in dorsal lithotomy position after adequate induction of general anesthesia. Levaquin 500 mg was given intravenously, preoperatively. Perineum and genitalia were prepped and draped in the usual sterile fashion. A #21 French cystourethroscope was inserted into the urethra, and the prostate was visualized. He did have some lateral lobe hyperplasia of the prostate, but otherwise no significant pathology in the urethra. The bladder was then entered and drained. Multiple bladder stones were seen and these were all less than half a centimeter apiece. The bladder stones were evacuated using cystoscope and irrigation with the Ellik evacuator. All stones were removed without difficulty. After the bladder was drained and all of the stones removed, the patient was awakened. He returned to the recovery room in satisfactory condition.

Abstract from Documentation:

During the cystoscopy, from which location were stones removed? **Bladder**

Time to Code:

Index: Cystourethroscopy, Removal, Calculus

Code: 52310 Cystourethroscopy with removal calculus from bladder

Case Study #7

Operative Report

Preoperative Diagnosis: A 6-mm stone in the left lower pole.

Postoperative Diagnosis: A 6-mm stone in the left lower pole.

Operation Performed: Left extracorporeal shockwave lithotripsy.

Anesthesia: Intravenous sedation.

Indications for Procedure: This is a 57-year-old man who has been known to have a stone in the left upper pole for a number of years. He recently presented with left renal colic. An X-ray showed the stone to have migrated into the proximal ureter. Recently, he underwent cystoscopy, the stone was successfully flushed into the kidney, and a double-J stent was placed. He now needs to be treated with ESWL.

Description of Procedure: The patient was placed onto the treatment table and, after the administration of intravenous sedation, he was positioned over the shockwave electrode. The X-ray showed the stone to now be located in the lower pole of the left kidney. Biaxial fluoroscopy was utilized to position the stone at the focal point of the shockwave generator. The stone was initially treated at 17 kV, increasing up to 24 kV. The stone was treated with 3000 shocks. Throughout the procedure, fluoroscopic manipulations and adjustments were made in order to maintain the stone in the focal point of the shockwave generator. At the conclusion of the procedure, the stone appeared to have fragmented nicely, and the patient was placed on a stretcher and taken to the recovery room in good condition.

Index: Lithotripsy, Kidney

Code: 50590 Lithotripsy, extracorporeal shock wave

Case Study #8

Operative Report

Preoperative Diagnosis: Urethral caruncle
Urethral stenosis

Postoperative Diagnosis: Same

Operative Procedure: Cystoscopy
External urethroplasty with excision of caruncle

Procedure: The patient is brought to the Cystoscopy Suite where general anesthesia is induced and maintained in the usual fashion. The patient is then placed in the dorsal lithotomy position. The external genitalia are prepped and draped in routine fashion. A 21 French panendoscope is assembled and inserted into the bladder without difficulty. Inspection of the urethra and bladder is carried out with both the straight and the right-angled lenses. The urethra is highly stenotic, and it has been difficult to pass the scope; however, it can pop through which caused some bleeding. There is a large caruncle protruding from the urethra, which has been very bothersome for the patient. The urethral mucosa more proximally is normal and bladder neck is normal. The trigone shows significant droppage. The ureteral orifices are identified. The urine efflux is clear from both sides. The orifices are normal in configuration. The remainder of the bladder wall is unremarkable, with no evidence for foreign body of tumor anywhere on the mucosa. Bladder capacity appears about normal.

Following cystoscopy, the urethral caruncle is grasped and then completely excised. An 18 French Foley catheter is inserted into the patient's bladder. Incision into the urethra is made at the 3 o'clock and 9 o'clock positions. Some additional mucosa in the 12 o'clock position is also excised. The Bovie cautery is used to control bleeding. The urethral catheter is removed, and inspection reveals that the urethra is somewhat closed and it is necessary to incise the urethra in the 12 o'clock position as well. Once this is done, fulguration controls the bleeding. The catheter is again removed, and inspection shows that now the urethra is wide open. There is no significant bleeding. The catheter is reinserted and will be left for drainage for several hours.

Following urethroplasty, the patient undergoes pelvic examination, which is unremarkable. The patient is taken to the recovery room in good condition.

Abstract from Documentation:

What procedures were performed through the endoscope? **Diagnostic only, no active surgical interventions.**

In addition to the endoscopy, what other procedures were performed?
Urethroplasty after incision to treat stricture

Excision of caruncle

Time to Code:

Index:

1. Cystourethroscopy

2. Urethroplasty, first stage

3. Excision, Lesion, Urethra

Codes:

52000–59 Cystourethroscopy—this code is identified as a "separate procedure." If a major procedure were performed, this code would not be assigned. In this case, the cystoscopy was a distinct procedure, which justifies use of modifier 59.

53400 Urethroplasty for stricture

53265 Excision urethral caruncle

Male Genital System Exercises

Medical Terminology Review

1. ____ epididymis (E)
2. ____ vas deferens (C)
3. ____ testicles (A)
4 ____ orchiectomy (B)
5. ____ circumcision (D)

A. organ that produces sperm

B. surgical removal of one or both testicles

C. duct that conveys sperm from testicles to urethra

D. surgical removal of foreskin

E. duct along which sperm passes to vas deferens

Case Studies

Case Study #1

Patient is a 55-year-old male with a Mentor inflatable three-piece penile prosthesis that had been causing problems. He was experiencing issues with prolonged erections while deflating the prosthesis. It was elected to remove the prosthesis and insert a Duraphase II penile prosthesis. There was some evidence of infection in the area, which was irrigated.

Index: Removal, Prosthesis, Penis

Code: 54411 Removal and replacement of all components of a multi-component inflatable penile prosthesis through an infected field at the same operative session, including irrigation and debridement of infected tissue.

Case Study #2

Operative Report

Preoperative Diagnosis: Left hydrocele

Postoperative Diagnosis: Same

Operation Performed: Left hydrocelectomy

Indications: This 55-year-old male with a history of left hydrocele swelling causing discomfort requesting intervention after evaluation and preoperative consultation.

Operation: Patient was sterilely prepped and draped in the usual fashion. A transverse incision across the left hemiscrotum was made approximately 4 cm in length down to the level of the hydrocele. Hydrocele was removed from the incision and stripped of its fibrous attachments. Hydrocele was opened and drained. The excess sac was removed and discarded. The sac was then everted with the testicle, and a running #2-0 chromic stitch in a locking fashion was placed across the edges of the sac. Meticulous hemostasis was achieved. The testicle and spermatic cord were then replaced back to the patient's left scrotum. There was no damage done to the vas deferens. The dartos layer was reapproximated using #2-0 running locking chromic stitch. The skin was closed in a running horizontal mattress fashion using #3-0 chromic. The patient tolerated the procedure well.

Abstract from Documentation:

Locate hydrocele in the Alphabetic Index. What documentation from the operative report is needed to accurately assign codes? **Unilateral vs. bilateral; if performed as an aspiration, or excision tunica vaginalis (covering over testis-scrotum) or of spermatic cord. In this case, tunica vaginalis.**

Time to Code:

Index: Hydrocele, Excision, Unilateral, Tunica Vaginalis

Code: 55040 Excision of Hydrocele, unilateral

Case Study #3

Operative Report

Procedure: Circumcision.

Description of Procedure: The patient was cleaned and draped in sterile fashion and was first numbed at the base of the penis with 1% lidocaine without epinephrine, after which time it was noted that the meatus was at the tip of the penis. The dorsum of the foreskin was then clamped, and an incision was made along the clamp line. The foreskin was then retracted; Gomco bell, size #2, was placed over the tip of the penis, and the foreskin was retracted over the bell and secured with a safety pin. The clamp was then placed and secured. It was held for approximately 5 minutes until appropriate blanching was obtained. The foreskin was then removed with a #11 blade. The Gomco bell and clamp were then removed. There was minimal bleeding. The patient was then dressed with a sterile Vaseline gauze, and the Betadine was also cleaned from the area. He was returned to the newborn nursery, fairly quiet, for observation. The mother was spoken with after the procedure and told that the patient tolerated it well, and she was satisfied.

Abstract from Documentation:

Refer to Circumcision in the Alphabetic Index. What information do you need from the operative report to begin your coding assignment selection process?

Technique: Repair, surgical excision or with Clamp and age (Newborn or not)

Time to Code:

Index: Circumcision, with Clamp, Newborn

Code: 54150 Circumcision using clamp

Case Study #4

Operative Report

Preoperative Diagnosis: Elevated prostate specific antigen

Postoperative Diagnosis: Same

Procedure Performed: Ultrasound-guided prostate needle biopsy

Anesthesia: General anesthesia

Complications: None

Specimens Removed: Twelve core needle biopsies of the prostate

Indications: The patient is a 57-year-old man. He was found on recent labs to have an elevated PSA at the level of 4.5. He was therefore consented for prostate needle biopsy.

Details of Procedures: Patient was brought back to the Cysto Suite and moved into the lateral decubitus position. After smooth induction of general anesthesia, a digital rectal exam was performed. There were no nodules palpated. The prostate was smooth, firm, and benign feeling. The ultrasound probe was then inserted into the rectum. There were no abnormalities seen on ultrasound. We then proceeded to take a total of 12 core needle specimens of the prostate, two from the right base, two from the right mid, two from the right apex, followed by two from the left base, two from left mid and two from the left apex. The patent tolerated the procedure well. There was minimal blood loss. Patient was transferred back to the Postanesthesia Care Unit in stable condition. He will be sent home with three days of antibiotics, and we will follow upon his pathology.

Time to Code:

Index: Biopsy, Prostate

Code: 55700 Biopsy, prostate; needle or punch, single or multiple, any approach

Case Study #5

Operative Report

Preoperative Diagnosis: T2C, NX, M0 prostate cancer

Postoperative Diagnosis: T2C, NX, M0 prostate cancer

Operation: Radical retropubic prostatectomy with bilateral pelvic lymph node dissection

Indications: This 62-year-old man had an elevated PSA of 12.5 on routine screening. He recently underwent a transrectal ultrasound and biopsy that revealed approximately 9 out of 10 cores positive for adenocarcinoma of the prostate. With hormonal therapy, his PSA preoperatively had decreased to 0.1 on androgen blockade.

Procedure: After administration of general anesthesia, the patient was placed in supine position, prepped, and draped in the usual sterile fashion. A midline incision was made to the left of the umbilicus and carried down to the public bone. The fascia was split in the midline as well as the rectus muscle, and the retropubic space was then entered. Each obturator fossa was delineated using blunt dissection. A fixed Balfour retractor was then placed.

A left pelvic lymph node dissection was then performed in the usual fashion. Care was taken to preserve the obturator nerve. It was noted that there were no grossly enlarged nodes in the area. Clips were used to control bleeding and lymph drainage.

A similar dissection was performed on the right side with no damage to the obturator nerve, and there were no grossly enlarged lymph nodes.

Frozen section analysis did not reveal any adenocarcinoma.

The endopelvic fascia was then identified and defatted. It was split along its lateral borders from the puboprostatic ligaments and down to the bladder neck. The dorsal vein complex and endopelvic fascia were then gathered using a curved Babcock clamp. Two 0 Vicryl suture ligatures were placed at the bladder neck to control bleeding.

A clamp was then passed between the anterior urethra and dorsal vein complex, and a 0 Vicryl suture was then tied around this complex. A second 0 Vicryl suture ligature was also placed in the most distal portion. The dorsal vein complex was divided using electrocautery, and excellent hemostasis was noted. The prostatic apex was identified with further sharp and blunt dissection.

The anterior half of the urethra was divided sharply using the #15 blade. Next, the Foley catheter was passed into the wound and divided. The posterior urethra was then sharply transected in a similar fashion. The catheter was used to provide some subtle traction of the prostate. The rectourethralis was taken down using a right-angle clamp and electrocautery. Each neurovascular bundle was also tied and ligated.

The prostate could be mobilized up to the bladder neck.

The lateral pedicles were controlled using 2-0 Vicryl sutures and divided. A small horizontal incision was then made over the seminal vesicles and ampulla of the vas. Each of these structures was then dissected out using sharp and blunt dissection. Clips were used to control bleeding. The seminal vesicles could be removed in their entirety. Each vas was clipped and ligated.

An anatomic bladder-neck-preserving dissection was then performed, and the prostate was sharply transected off the bladder neck. The bladder mucosa was everted using a running 4-0 Monocryl suture. Two 0 Vicryl sutures were placed at the 6 o'clock position to tighten the bladder neck to 20 French.

Four 2-0 Monocryl sutures were placed in this bladder neck at equally spaced distances. A Greenwald sound was then placed into the distal urethral stump and the corresponding bladder neck sutures were then placed into the urethral stump under direct visualization.

The bladder neck was then brought down to the urethral stump using a curved Babcock clamp. All bleeding was controlled and the wound was irrigated with normal saline. The anastomosis was then tied down and, upon testing, was shown to be watertight.

Two Jackson-Pratt drains were then brought out through each lower abdominal quadrant in a separate stab wound incision. They were used to drain each obturator fossa and around the anastomosis. The fascia was reapproximated using interrupted #1 figure-of-eight Vicryl sutures. The subcutaneous tissue was closed with a running 2-0 chromic suture. The skin was reapproximated using staples. Each drain was sutured in with a 2-0 silk suture. The patient tolerated the procedure well and was discharged to the recovery room in stable condition.

Abstract from Documentation:

Review the Alphabetic Index for the coding selection for Prostatectomy. What documentation would be needed to choose the range to verify? **Laparoscopic, Perineal, Retropubic, Suprapubic or Transurethral**

Also, for perineal/retropubic and suprapubic, must determine if the procedure was partial or radical.

Time to Code:

Index: Prostatectomy, Retropubic, Radical (55840–55845, 55866)

Code: 55845 Prostatectomy, retropubic radical, with or without nerve sparing; with bilateral pelvic lymphadenectomy

Female Genital System Exercises

Medical Terminology Review

1. ____ cervix (D)
2. ____ vagina (C)
3. ____ ovary (B)
4. ____ colposcopy (E)
5. ____ laparoscopy (A)

A. surgical procedure; instrument inserted into abdominal wall to view internal organs

B. produces eggs

C. tube leading from genitalia to cervix

D. passage forming lower end of uterus

E. surgical procedure to examine vagina and cervix

Case Studies

Case Study #1

Operative Note: Patient treated for a 2.5 cm lesion of vagina. The lesion was lasered and hemostasis obtained for bleeding. Specimens sent to pathology for evaluation.

Index: (Laser is a form of destruction.)

Lesion, vagina, destruction (results in code 57061)

Code: 57061 Destruction of vaginal lesion(s)

Case Study #2

The OB/GYN physician delivers a baby via cesarean section. The physician has provided all obstetrical care prior to delivery and will continue to follow the patient for her postpartum care.

Abstract from Documentation:

What coding guidelines pertain to maternity care and are applicable in this case? **Code 59510 would be reported by a physician providing global care for a cesarean delivery.**

Time to Code:

Index: Cesarean Delivery, Routine Care

Code: 59510 Routine obstetric care including antepartum care, cesarean delivery, and postpartum care

Case Study #3

Operative Note: The patient is a 59-year-old Gravida 3, Para 3, who was experiencing postmenopausal bleeding for the last five months and her evaluation included a normal endometrial biopsy. The patient also was found to have a right adnexal mass on CAT scan confirmed with ultrasound, as well as a small cystic mass in the left ovary. Given the patient's age and despite a normal CA-125, the need for surgical evaluation of the complex adnexal mass was discussed. The patient also preferred a total abdominal hysterectomy to be performed because of postmenopausal bleeding and to see a definitive diagnosis and treatment of that condition. Informed consent was obtained for hysterectomy and bilateral salpingo-oophorectomy.

Abstract from Documentation:

Review the Alphabetic Index for the selection under the term Hysterectomy. What documentation is needed to locate a coding selection? How it was performed (abdominal, vaginal, supracervical, laparoscopic). Further documentation includes total vs. radical.

Time to Code:

Index: Hysterectomy, Abdominal, Total (58150, 58200, 58956)

Code: **58150 Total abdominal hysterectomy with or without removal of tubes and ovaries**

Case Study #4

Operative Note

This 74-year-old woman underwent a partial vulvectomy 6 months ago for carcinoma in situ. She now was found to have recurrent disease of her vulva and a partial vulvectomy was performed. The skin was dissected towards the introitus and the posterior vagina was dissected for approximately 1 inch into the proximal vagina. The vaginal mucosa was undermined for at least 2 cm and approximated to the perineal skin by interrupted 2-0 Vicryl sutures. The anterior vulva lesion was then excised with a margin of approximately 0.5 cm. The lesion itself was approximately 2 cm in diameter. Bleeding points were cauterized. Wounds closed with interrupted 3-0 Vicryl.

Pathology Report

Specimens: vulva lesion with anal margin, anterior vulva, periurethral

Abstract from Documentation:

Review the Alphabetic Index for coding selections for vulvectomy procedures. What documentation is needed for the coding selection? Complete, Partial, Radical, Simple

Note the definitions for simple, radical, partial and complete vulvectomy codes (listed before code 56405). What documentation from this operative note leads you to the correct definition?

Physician dictates that the vulvectomy was partial (removes less than 80% of vulvar area). Was this a *radical* (removal of skin and deep subcutaneous tissue) or *simple* (removal of skin and superficial subcutaneous tissue) procedure? The term undermined (dig beneath) implies that it was beyond the superficial subcutaneous tissues. To be safe, a coder may want to query the physician.

Time to Code:

Index: Vulvectomy, partial (56620, 56630–56632)

Code: **56630 Vulvectomy, radical, partial**

Case Study #5

Operative Note: Patient has chronic complaints of right pelvic pain. Taken to OR for a laparoscopy. Inspection into the pelvis revealed multiple adhesions attached to the left tube and ovary. These adhesions were lysed bluntly with probe. No other abnormalities noted.

> **Index: Laparoscopy, Lysis of Adhesions**
>
> **Code: 58660 Laparoscopy, surgical; with lysis of adhesions**

Case Study #6

Preoperative Diagnosis: Dysfunctional uterine bleeding

Postoperative Diagnosis: Same

Operations: ThermaChoice balloon endometrial ablation

Procedure: The patient was taken to the OR and under adequate anesthesia; she was prepped and draped in the dorsolithotomy position for a vaginal procedure. The Therma-Choice system was assembled and primed. The catheter with the balloon was placed inside the endometrial cavity and slowly filled with fluid until it stabilized at a pressure of approximately 175 to 180 mm Hg. The system was then preheated and after preheating to 87 degrees C. eight minutes of therapeutic heat was applied to the lining of the endometrium. The fluid was allowed to drain from the balloon, and the system was removed. The procedure was discontinued.

> **Index: Ablation, endometrial (results in code 58353)**
>
> **Code: 58353 Endometrial ablation, thermal, without hysteroscopic guidance**

Case Study #7

Operative Report

Preoperative Diagnosis: Perimenopausal bleeding. Possible endometrial hypoplasia.

Postoperative Diagnosis: Perimenopausal bleeding

Procedures: Hysteroscopy. Dilatation and curettage

Specimen to Lab: Endometrial curetting

Estimated Bloods Loss: Less than 5 mL

Description of Procedure: The patient was taken to the operating room and under satisfactory general anesthesia was examined, noted to have a normal-size uterus. No adnexal masses noted. She was prepped and draped in the routine fashion, the speculum placed in the vagina, and the anterior lip of the cervix grasped with a single-tooth tenaculum. The uterus sounded to 8 cm and easily admitted a #21 K-Pratt, so no further dilation was necessary. A 12-degree hysteroscope was placed, using lactated Ringer as the distending medium, and the cervical canal was normal. The cavity revealed just fronds of tissue. There was tissue sticking out that did not have a particularly polypoid appearance. No other lesions could be appreciated that were polypoid. Curettage with a Milan curette and a serrated curette and then polyp forceps being introduced revealed minimal tissue, and 1 piece of tissue of 5 mm that might be consistent with what was seen on previous sonogram. The hysteroscope was then replaced. No other lesions could be appreciated, and the walls appeared smooth. At this time the hysteroscope was removed, and the tenaculum removed. The tenaculum site was touched with silver nitrate. The bleeding was minimal at the end of the procedure. She was taken to the recovery room in satisfactory condition.

Abstract from Documentation:

> ***What procedures were performed?*** **Hysteroscopy, D&C, removal of tissue (curette)**
>
> ***Refer to coding textbook, what guidelines pertain to this case?*** **No additional code is assigned to identify D&C when performed with hysteroscopy.**

Time to Code:

Index: **Hysteroscopy, Surgical with Biopsy**

Code: **58558 Hysteroscopy, surgical; with sampling of endometrium and/or polypectomy, with or without D&C**

Case Study #8

Operative Report

Preoperative Diagnosis: Desire for sterilization

Postoperative Diagnosis: Desire for sterilization

Procedure: Postpartum tubal ligation

Procedure in Detail: The patient was taken to the operating room with an IV line in place. She was placed on the operating room table and a 1.5 cm incision was made in the inferior fold of the umbilicus, continued through the subcutaneous tissue, rectus fascia, and parietal peritoneum as the incision was tracked ventrally using Allis clamps. Peritoneum was entered without difficulty. There was no evidence of vessel damage. Retractors were placed in the incision. At first, the left tube was visualized, grasped with a Babcock clamp, and pulled into the operative field. A hemostat was placed in an avascular plane of mesosalpinx, and a segment of tube was isolated and tied off using 2-0 plain gut. The segment was dissected and handed off the field. Pedicles were bovied. No active bleeding was noted. This was repeated on the opposite side.

Fascia and peritoneum were closed together using running continuous interlocking sutures of 0 Vicryl on a cutting needle. The wound was dressed and the patient taken to recovery in good condition.

Abstract from Documentation:

Refer to the key term in the Alphabetic Index. What information is needed to assign a CPT code for this procedure? **If it was performed laparoscopically or not**

Time to Code:

Index: **Tubal Ligation 58600**

Code: **58600 Ligation or transection of fallopian tube(s) abdominal or vaginal approach, unilateral or bilateral**

Case Study #9

Operative Report

Preoperative Diagnosis: Uterine fibroids

Postoperative Diagnosis: Multiple uterine fibroids, uterus –250 g, 2 cm right ovarian cyst

Procedure: Laparoscopic-assisted vaginal hysterectomy with bilateral salpingo-oophorectomy

Procedure in Detail: The patient was taken to the operating room and placed in the supine position. After adequate general anesthesia had been obtained, the patient was prepped and draped in the usual fashion for laparoscopic-assisted vaginal hysterectomy. The bladder was drained. A small infraumbilical skin incision was made with the scalpel, and 10 mm laparoscopic sleeve and trocar were introduced without difficulty. The trocar was removed. The laparoscope was placed and 2 L of CO_2 gas was insufflated in the patient's abdomen.

A second incision was made suprapubically and a 12-mm laparoscopic sleeve and trocar were introduced under direct visualization. A 5-mm laparoscopic sleeve and trocar were placed in the left lower quadrant under direct visualization. A manipulator was used to examine the patient's pelvic organs.

There was a small cyst on the right ovary. Both ovaries were free from adhesions. The ureters were free from the operative field. After measuring the ovarian distal pedicles, the endo-GIA staple was placed across each round ligament.

At this time, attention was turned to the vaginal part of the procedure. A weighted speculum was placed in the vagina. The anterior lip of the cervix was grasped with a Lahey tenaculum. Posterior colpotomy incision was made and the posterior peritoneum entered in this fashion. The uterosacral ligaments were bilaterally clamped, cut and Heaney sutured with #1 chromic. The cardinal ligaments were bilaterally clamped, cut and ligated. The anterior vaginal mucosa was then incised with the scalpel, and with sharp and blunt dissection, the bladder was freed from the underlying cervix. The bladder pillars were bilaterally clamped, cut and ligated. The uterine vessels were then bilaterally clamped, cut and ligated. Visualization was difficult because the patient had a very narrow pelvic outlet. In addition, several small fibroids made placement of clamps somewhat difficult. Using the clamp, cut and tie method, after the anterior peritoneum had been entered with scissors, the uterus was then left without vascular supply. The fundus was delivered by flipping the uterus posteriorly; and through an avascular small pedicle, Heaney clamps were placed across; and the uterus was then removed en bloc with the tubes and ovaries attached.

At this point, the remaining Heaney pedicles were ligated with a free-hand suture of 0 chromic. Sponge and instrument counts were correct. Avascular pedicles were inspected and found to be hemostatic. The posterior vaginal cuff was then closed using running interlocking suture of #1 chromic. The anterior peritoneum was then grasped, and using pursestring suture of 0 chromic, the peritoneum was closed. The vaginal cuff was then closed reincorporating the previously tagged uterosacral ligaments into the vaginal cuff through the anterior and posterior vaginal cuff. Another figure-of-eight suture totally closed the cuff. Hemostasis was excellent. Foley was then placed in the patient's bladder and clear urine was noted to be draining. At the point, the laparoscope was placed back through the 10-mm sleeve and the vaginal cuff inspected. A small amount of old blood was suctioned away, but all areas were hemostatic.

The laparoscopic instruments were removed after the excess gas had been allowed to escape. The incisions were closed first with suture of 2-0 Vicryl through the fascia of each incision, and then the skin edges were reapproximated with interrupted sutures of 3-0 plain. Sponge and instrument counts were correct. The patient was awakened from general anesthesia and taken to the recovery room in stable condition.

Abstract from Documentation:

Refer to the key term Hysterectomy in the Alphabetic Index. What key documentation is needed to lead to the correct coding range? Vaginal and then Laparoscopic drives the coding range. After the range of codes is identified and verified, other key documentation is needed (e.g. size of uterus, removal of tubes and ovaries).

Time to Code:

Index: **Hysterectomy, Vaginal, Removal Tubes/Ovaries**

Code: **58552 Laparoscopic, surgical, with vaginal hysterectomy, for uterus 250 g or less with removal of tube(s) and ovary(s)**

Nervous System Exercises

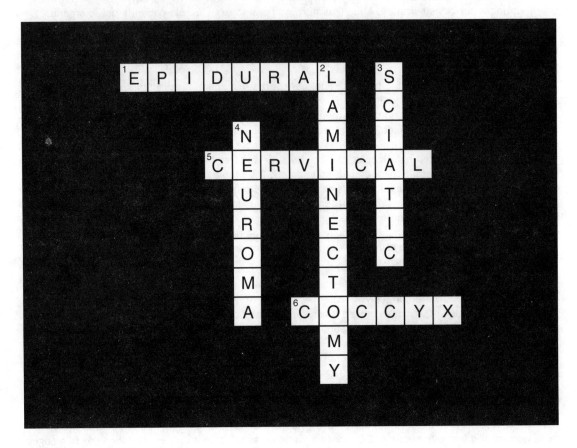

Across

1. Space around dura mater in spinal cord [EPIDURAL]
5. Vertebra of neck [CERVICAL]
6. Base of spine [COCCYX]

Down

2. Surgical removal of vertebrae [LAMINECTOMY]
3. Major nerve runs back of thigh [SCIATIC]
4. Tumor of nerves [NEUROMA]

Case Studies

Case Study #1

Operative Note for Cervical Epidural Injection: Patient has been experiencing neck pain for several years. Using fluoroscopic guidance, an epidural needle is inserted into the epidural space. A combination of an anesthetic and cortisone steroid solution is injected into the epidural space.

Abstract from Documentation:

Refer to Basic CPT/HCPCS for guidance on coding for spinal injections. What documentation is needed for coding selection? **Site of injection and substance (site is cervical, substance is anesthetic and steroid). Useful website: http://www.spine-health.com**

Time to Code:

Index: Injection, Spinal Cord, Anesthetic 62310–62319

Code: 62310 Injection, single, (including anesthetic, steroid); cervical

Case Study #2

Preoperative Diagnosis: Spinal cord stimulator battery replacement

Postoperative Diagnosis: Spinal cord stimulator battery replacement

Operation Performed: Removal of spinal cord stimulator batteries and replacement with new batteries

No complications

No specimens

Indications for Surgery: Patient is a 67-year-old man who had spinal cord stimulator implanted approximately five years ago. He comes back because of lack of functioning in this system. Decision was made to proceed with removal of the old batteries and replacement with new one. The patient understands the risks and benefits of the procedure.

Description of Surgery: The patient was placed in supine position and the area where the batteries were located on the left side was prepped and draped in the sterile fashion. The patient was infiltrated with lidocaine 1%. It was reopened with a #15 blade, and then the batteries were removed from the pocket and disconnected from the lead wires. A new battery system was reconnected. Wound was closed with #3-0 Vicryl and staples for skin.

Abstract from Documentation:

What is a spinal cord stimulator? **Also called neurostimulator, it is an implantable device often used to treat chronic pain. The pulse generator holds the batteries; therefore, replacement of batteries codes as replacement of pulse generator.**

Time to Code:

Index: Replacement, Neurostimulator, Pulse Generator/Receiver, Spinal

Code: 63685 Insertion or replacement of spinal neurostimulator pulse generator

Case Study #3

Operative Note: Patient has lumbar stenosis at L3-4 and L4-5. Performed a right partial L3 and partial L4 hemilaminectomy with undermining laminotomy for decompression of nerve roots.

> **Index: Hemilaminectomy 63020–63044**
>
> **Codes:**
>> **63030 Laminotomy (hemilaminectomy)—one interspace, lumbar**
>>
>> **63035 each additional interspace**

Case Study #4

Operative Report

Preoperative Diagnosis: Right carpal tunnel syndrome

Operation: Right carpal tunnel release

Indications: The patient is a 55-year-old man who has a history of right hand pain and numbness. He was found to have a right carpal tunnel syndrome by EMG. The patient has been treated conservatively without any improvements, so a decision was made to proceed with a release of the right carpal tunnel.

Description: The patient was placed supine on the operating table, where the right hand was anesthetized with lidocaine 1%. An incision was made with a #15 blade down to the ligament which was incised and was split with sharp scissors. The nerve was found to be completely free. The area was irrigated with antibiotic solution and then the area was closed with #3-0 Vicryl and #4-0 nylon for the skin.

> **Index: Carpal Tunnel Syndrome, decompression**
>
> **Code: 64721–RT Neuroplasty and/or transposition; median nerve at carpal tunnel**

Case Study #5

Operative Report

Preoperative Diagnosis: Left ulnar nerve entrapment at the elbow

Postoperative Diagnosis: Same

Procedure: Left ulnar nerve decompression at the elbow

Indications: The patient has a history of numbness in the fourth and fifth digits of the left hand and also some weakness in the grip. He complains of pain in the ulnar side of the left arm. He had an EMG which was positive for entrapment of the left ulnar nerve at the elbow and he had conservation treatment with some improvement of the mode of function, with severe significant numbness and pain. Because of the symptoms, the decision was made to proceed with a decompression of the left ulnar nerve at the elbow.

Description of Surgery: The patient was placed in supine position with the left hand on the surgical stand. The arm was then prepped, draped and then an incision was marked at the level of the left elbow. The incision was infiltrated with lidocaine 1% and then the incision was made with a #15 blade. With the use of bipolar coagulator, the bleeding was easily controlled and then the ulnar nerve was exposed at the level of the elbow proximally and distally. The ulnar nerve was completely compressed and was released from a dense scar. Antibiotic solution was used to irrigate the area and then the area was closed with #3-0 Vicryl and staples.

> **Index: Nerves, Decompression**
>
> **Code: 64718–LT Neuroplasty; ulnar nerve at elbow**

Case Study #6

Operative Report

Preoperative Diagnosis: Chronic intractable radicular pain

Postoperative Diagnosis: Chronic intractable radicular pain

Procedure: Placement of percutaneous spinal cord stimulator

Indications: This is a 54-year-old man with intractable back and particularly left leg pain for several years.

Details of Procedure: The patient was taken to OR and positioned on his right side. He was prepped with pHisoHex, and draped using a Vi-Drape. The skin was infiltrated with a mixture of 0.5% Marcaine and 2% lidocaine.

Using a 22-gauge spinal needle, the T12-L1 interspace was sought. After confirming this location on fluoroscopy, the needle was removed; and the Pyle needle was placed. Using radiological images, the Pyle needle was advanced to the epidural space. The Pisces Coag-Plus lead was passed through the needle into the epidural space. Under fluoroscopic guidance, the course of the electrode was monitored as the electrode was passed from the T11-T12 level to the T7 level. At this time, the electrodes were connected, and stimulation was undertaken. Next, the electrodes #2 and #3 were charged, with the #3 electrode getting the negative charge. The patient got excellent coverage of his left leg down below his knee and as far up as his lower back. He was very satisfied with the level and area of coverage. We were able to obtain satisfactory coverage at approximately 3 V with a pulse rate of 50 and a band width of 200. It was decided then to accept this positioning of the electrode, and the electrode was then taped to the patient's back using benzoin and Steri-Strips. Just prior to taping the electrode, the position was confirmed with X-ray. The patient was discharged to the recovery room in satisfactory condition

Index: Spinal Cord, Implantation, Electrode

Code: 63650 Percutaneous implantation of neurostimulator electrode array, epidural

Case Study #7

Operative Report

Preoperative Diagnosis: L5-S1 herniated disc on the left side

Postoperative Diagnosis: L5-S1 herniated disc on the left side

Operation: L5-S1 discectomy and L5 nerve root decompression

Indications for Surgery: The patient is a 53-year-old male who has a history of low back pain and left leg pain in the L5 distribution. An MRI shows the presence of a herniated disc at L5-S1 migrated up impinging the L5 nerve root on the left side. The patient has been treated conservatively without any improvement.

Description of Surgery: The patient was intubated and placed in prone position. Then an incision was marked on the lower back and was prepped and draped in sterile fashion. The incision was made with a #10 scalpel, Bovie coagulator and down to the fascia. At this point, the fascia was incised with a #15 blade. A flap of the fascia was then retracted with #2-0 Vicryl and the muscle was gently dissected and retracted with a Taylor retractor. Under the microscope, a curette was placed between the L5-S1 and X-rays were obtained. The X-rays showed that the curette was between L5 and S1 until under the microscope with microdissection, and with the use of a Midas Rex the lamina of L5 was partially drilled off and yellow ligament was opened, removed and then the L5 nerve root was identified. A large herniated disc was then found, removed and the L5 nerve root was completely decompressed. At this point, the interspace at L5-S1 was entered for the disc removed laterally, and then a complete decompression of the L5 into the foramen was accomplished. At this point, the area was irrigated with antibiotic solution and a paste of Depo-Medrol, Amicar and morphine was left in place. The fascia was closed with a #2-0 Vicryl, subcutaneous tissue with a #3-0 Vicryl, and the skin was closed with subcuticular #4-0 Vicryls.

Abstract from Documentation:

Refer to Basic CPT/HCPCS Coding for coding guidance. What is a discectomy?
A discectomy is a surgery done to remove a herniated disc from the spinal. A laminectomy is often involved to permit access to the intervertebral disc.

After the location of the curette was confirmed, what was the first surgical action?
Lamina was partially drilled off (hemilaminectomy).

Refer to this term in the Alphabetic Index.

Time to Code:

Index: Hemilaminectomy. 63020–63044

Code: 63030 Laminotomy (hemilaminectomy) with decompression of nerve root(s), including foraminotomy and/or excision of herniated intervertebral disc; one interspace, lumbar

An interactive video of this procedure can be found at: http://www.spine-health.com

Eye and Ocular Adnexa Exercises

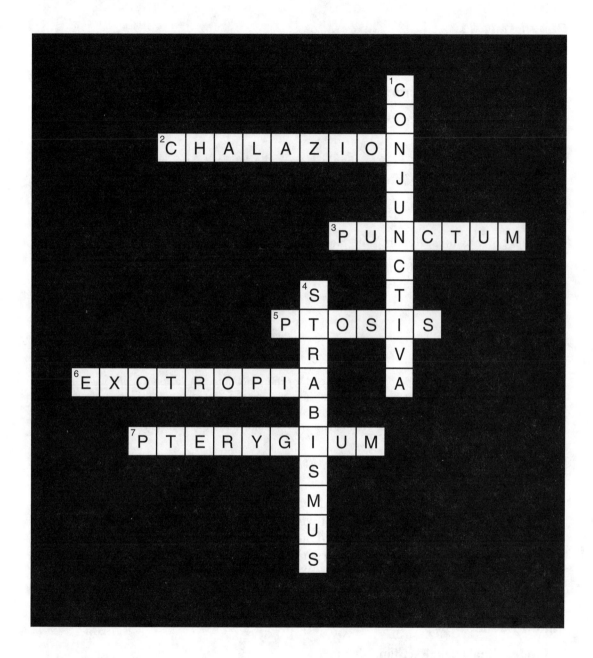

Across

2. Cyst of eyelid [CHALAZION]
3. Opening of tear duct [PUNCTUM]
5. Drooping of eyelids [PTOSIS]
6. Eyes deviate outward [EXOTROPIA]
7. Benign growth of conjunctiva [PTERYGIUM]

Down

1. Inner part of eyelid [CONJUNCTIVA]
4. Abnormal alignment of eyes [STRABISMUS]

Case Studies

Case Study #1

Patient diagnosed with exotropia. Surgeon performs bilateral recession of lateral rectus muscles.

Abstract from Documentation:

What is the definition of exotropia? **Type of strabismus in which the eyes are turned outward.**

Refer to Basic CPT/HCPCS textbook: How is the lateral rectus muscle classified (vertical or horizontal)? **Horizontal**

Time to Code:

Index: Strabismus, Repair, One Horizontal Muscle

Code: 67311–50 Strabismus surgery, recession or resection procedure; one horizontal muscle

Case Study #2

Operative Note: Chalazion incision and drainage of the right eye

Procedure: The right eye was prepped and draped for the procedure. Chalazion forceps were used to grasp the upper eyelid. The surface of the chalazion was incised. The contents of the chalazion were curetted. Chalazion forceps were removed. Hemostasis was achieved. Maxitrol ointment was placed in the eye with an overlying eye pad. The patient was transferred to the recovery area in stable condition.

Abstract from Documentation:

Refer to Chalazion in the Alphabetic Index. What documentation is needed to assign a correct CPT code? **Documentation of which eyelid, and whether multiple or single. Note that the operative note refers to incision and drainage and the subcategory is under the title of Excision and Destruction. Note that the physician "cut into the chalazion" and subsequently "curetted" the cyst. The technique described is similar to excision.**

Time to Code:

Index: Chalazion, Excision, Single

Code: 67800–RT Excision of chalazion; single

Case Study #3

Operative Report

Preoperative Diagnosis: Dermatochalasis of bilateral upper eyelids

Postoperative Diagnosis: Dermatochalasis of bilateral upper eyelids

Operation: Bilateral upper lid blepharoplasty

Indications: Patient is a 41-year-old female with a history of progressive upper eyelid hooding related to her redundant skin. The patient complains that this makes her eyelids feel heavy and interferes with her vision, particularly when she is tired. Patient was seen in the Outpatient Clinic and offered bilateral upper lid blepharoplasty.

Details: Patient brought to the operating room and placed on the operating table in supine position. After adequate intravenous sedation had been obtained, the patient's upper eyelids were marked for incision and infiltrated with 5 cc of 0.5% lidocaine mixed with 1:300,000 epinephrine in each lid. The patient's face and head were prepped and draped in the standard operative fashion. The previously marked bilateral upper lids were incised through the skin and the orbicularis muscle using #15 surgical blade. The marked segment was excised sharply with #15 surgical blade with adequate tension on the operative field. The excision was carried down through the muscle and the fat layer was easily visible. This procedure was repeated identically on the opposite lid. Next, the middle fat pad, which was readily identifiable, was gently teased out with a concave applicator and forceps and the pad was removed with the Bovie cautery. Next, the medial fat pad was also dissected out using gentle blunt dissection. The fat pat was retracted into the field and removed using the electrocautery. The procedure was repeated identically on the opposite lid. The operative field was then examined for hemostasis. The electrocautery was used to dry up any small bleeders. The wound was closed in a single layer using interrupted #6-0 Ethibond sutures. The wounds were dressed with Bacitracin and iced moist gauze and the patient was transferred to the recovery room in stable condition.

Abstract from Documentation:

Refer to the key operative term in the Alphabetic Index and note the code range.

What documentation is needed from the record to correctly assign a CPT code(s)? **Note whether the procedure was performed on the upper or lower eyelids (unilateral or bilateral). Next, note that the diagnostic information contributes to the coding in this case (excessive skin weighting down lid).**

Important to note that that the blepharoplasty codes appear in the Integumentary System section. More extensive eyelid repair codes appear in the Eye and Ocular Adnexa section (e.g. 67901).

Time to Code:

Index: Blepharoplasty 15820–15823

Code: 15823–50 Blepharoplasty; upper eyelid; with excessive skin weighting down lid

Case Study #4

Operative Note

Pterygium removal with conjunctival graft

Procedure Details: Local anesthesia was achieved with a 50/50 mixture of 2% lidocaine and 0.75% bupivacaine with hyaluronidase.. The eye was prepped and draped in the usual sterile fashion. The lashes were isolated on Steri-Strips and the lids separated with the wire speculum. The pterygium was marked with a marking pen and subconjunctival injection of 1% lidocaine with epinephrine was injected underneath the pterygium. The pterygium was then resected and the body of the pterygium was resected with sharp dissection with Westcott scissors. The head of the pterygium was dissected off the cornea with Martinez corneal dissector. The cornea was then smoothed with an ototome bur. Hemostasis was achieved with bipolar cautery.

A conjunctival graft measuring 10 × 8 mm was harvested from the superior bulbar conjunctiva by marking the area, injecting it with subconjunctival 1% lidocaine with epinephrine. This was dissected with Westcott scissors and sutured in place with multiple interrupted 9-0 Dexon sutures. Subconjunctival Decadron and gentamicin injections were given. A bandage contact lens was placed on the eye. Maxitrol ointment was placed on the eye. A patch was placed on the eye. The patient tolerated the procedure well and was taken to the recovery room in good condition.

Index: Pterygium, Excision, with Graft

Code: 65426 Excision or transposition or pterygium; with graft

Case Study #5

Operative Note

Patient has possible nasolacrimal duct obstruction.

Procedure: Nasolacrimal duct probing and irrigation for right eye

Procedure Details: The patient was brought into the operating room. The operative eye was prepped and draped. A punctal dilator was used to dilate the superior and inferior puncta of the operative eye. A double-0 Bowman probe was passed through one of the puncta and passed into the common canaliculus. The probe was passed into the nasolacrimal sac and down the bony canal of the nasolacrimal duct. The probe was passed into the nasal cavity beneath the inferior turbinate. The probe was removed. A lacrimal cannula attached to a 3-cc syringe filled with fluorescein solution was used to cannulate the nasolacrimal duct. An aspirating catheter was placed in the ipsilateral nasal cavity. Fluorescein was irrigated into the nasolacrimal duct. Fluorescein was aspirated from the nasal cavity following the irrigation. This demonstrated patency of the nasolacrimal drainage system. The lacrimal cannula and aspiration catheter were removed. The patient tolerated the procedure well and was transferred to the recovery room in stable condition.

Abstract from Documentation:

What documentation is needed to assign the correct CPT code? **If the procedure required general anesthesia or probing included insertion of tube or stent or balloon catheter dilation**

Time to Code:

Index: Nasolacrimal Duct, Exploration

Code: 68810–RT Probing of nasolacrimal duct, with or without irrigation

Case Study #6

Emergency Department Record

Patient brought to the ED from work with complaints of a foreign body in the right eye. He was wearing safety glasses but stated a piece of metal flew in the eye. He reports slight irritation but no blurred vision. PERLA: Fundi without edema. There was no foreign body on lid eversion. Slit lamp shows a foreign body approximately 2 to 3 o'clock on the edge of the cornea. It appears to be metallic. Iris is intact. There are no cells in the anterior chamber.

Procedure: Two drops of Alcaine were used in the right eye. With use of slit lamp, foreign body was removed without difficulty.

Impression: Residual corneal abrasion

Disposition: Foreign body removed from right eye

Index: Removal, Foreign Body, Cornea with Slit Lamp

Code: 65222–RT Removal of foreign body, external eye; corneal, with slit lamp

Auditory System Exercises

Medical Terminology Review

1. ____ myringotomy (C)
2. ____ tympanoplasty (E)
3. ____ stapedectomy (D)
4. ____ Eustachian tube (A)
5. ____ tympanum (B)

A. connects middle ear with nasopharynx

B. eardrum

C. surgical incision into eardrum

D. surgical removal of innermost chain of 3 ossicles in middle ear

E. surgical repair of middle ear

Case Studies

Case Study #1

Physician Office Note: Examination of the ear canal on both sides revealed impacted cerumen, tightly on the right side and a little bit on the left. With the use of ear curet, the impacted cerumen was removed. Both ears were irrigated with saline solution and suctioned dry to clean out all the debris.

Index: Cerumen, Removal

Code: 69210 Removal of impacted cerumen, one or both ears (No need for modifier because the description states "one or both".)

Case Study #2

Operative Report

Preoperative Diagnosis: Recurrent otitis media with persistent bilateral middle ear effusion

Postoperative Diagnosis: Same

Procedure: Bilateral myringotomy with ventilating tube insertion

Procedure in Detail: The patient was prepped and draped in the usual fashion under general anesthesia. Myringotomy was performed in the anterior-inferior quadrant and thick fluid suctioned from the middle ear space. A Type I Paparella tube was then inserted. Then a myringotomy was performed on the left ear, again thick fluid was suctioned from the middle ear space. A Type I Paparella tube was then inserted. Cortisporin Otic Suspension drops were then placed in both ear canals and cotton in the ears. The patient was awakened and returned to the recovery room in satisfactory condition.

Abstract from Documentation:

Refer to *Basic CPT/HCPCS* for guidelines pertaining to myringotomy for insertion of tubes.

Time to Code:

Index: Tympanostomy 69433–69436

Code: 69436–50 Tympanostomy (requiring insertion of ventilating tube), general anesthesia

Case Study #3

Operative Report

Preoperative Diagnosis: Left tympanic membrane perforation

Postoperative Diagnosis: Left tympanic membrane perforation

Procedure: Left tympanoplasty

Indications for Operation: This patient is a man who sustained a tympanic membrane perforation 20 years ago after diving into a pool. He has now sought repair.

Details of Operation: After induction of anesthesia, the table was rotated 180 degrees, and the left ear was prepped and draped in sterile fashion. Operating microscope was then used to inspect the left ear. A large central perforation encompassing approximately 50% of the tympanic membrane was visualized. Malleus was clearly visualized and appeared intact. Using 1% lidocaine with 1:1000 epinephrine injection, four quadrant canal injection was performed. Next, the patient was rotated away and a postauricular incision was made. Temporalis fascia was harvested and kept aside. A T-shaped incision was made on soft tissue and Lempert elevator was used to elevate the canal walls again. A freer was used to elevate the canal walls again and the previously made canal wall incisions were identified. The vascular flap was then raised. Canal wall skin was elevated to the level of the annulus, which was then elevated. The middle ear space was entered through the mucosa using a Rosen. The chorda tympani nerve was identified and preserved. The tympanic membrane was then raised off the chorda tympani nerve and the malleus. Gelfoam was placed in the anterior most aspect of the middle ear space, and the fascia was then laid into place. Tympanic membrane was laid down over the fascia. The vascular flap was then laid back down and the postauricular incision was closed with Vicryl sutures. PSO ointment was applied to the middle ear space and at this point, the left ear was cleaned. Sterile dressing was then placed over the ear and the patient was returned to the recovery room.

Abstract from Documentation:

Refer to Tympanoplasty in the Alphabetic Index. What types of documentation should be searched for when reading the operative report? **Were other procedures performed, such as mastoidectomy, ossicular chain reconstruction, etc.? Note the entry for "without mastoidectomy".**

Time to Code:

Index: Tympanoplasty, without Mastoidectomy

Codes:

69631–LT Tympanoplasty without mastoidectomy (including canal plasty, atticotomy and/or middle ear surgery), initial or revision; without ossicular chain reconstruction

69990 Operating Microscope

Case Study #4

Operative Report

Preoperative Diagnosis: Conductive hearing loss, right ear

Postoperative Diagnosis: Conductive hearing loss, right ear

Operation: Stapedectomy

Procedure: The patient was prepped and draped in the usual manner. The external auditory canal wall was injected with 1% lidocaine and 1:100,000 epinephrine. The tympanomeatal flap was elevated using a vertical rolling knife. The middle ear was entered and chorda tympani nerve identified and annulus lifted out of the tympanic sulcus. After elevating the tympanomeatal flap anteriorly, the ossicles were palpated and the malleus and incus moved freely and the stapes was fixed. The posterior superior canal wall was curetted down after mobilizing the chorda tympani nerve, which was left intact. The stapes footplate was easily visualized and found to be markedly thickened. The pyramidal process was identified and the stapes tendon cut, and an IS joint knife was used to dislocate the joint between the incus and stapes. Next, a small and a large Buckingham mirror were used along with a drill to drill out the stapes footplate. After this was done, a .5 × 4-mm Schuknecht piston prosthesis was placed in position. Crimping was achieved, and there was an excellent fit, and the stapes footplate area was then packed with small pieces of Gelfoam. The tympanomeatal flap was then put back in proper position, and the middle ear was then packed with rayon strips of Cortisporin and a cotton ball in the middle to form a rosette. The patient was awakened in the operating room and transferred to recovery in no apparent distress.

Index: Stapes, Excision, with Footplate Drill Out

Code: 69661–RT Stapedectomy or stapedotomy with reestablishment of ossicular continuity, with or without use of foreign material; with footplate drill out

Chapter 5
Radiology

Medical Terminology Review

1. ____ CT Scan (B)
2. ____ Nuclear Medicine (E)
3. ____ MRI (C)
4. ____ Ultrasound (D)
5. ____ X-ray (A)

A. uses electromagnetic radiation to make images

B. creates multiple images with computer technology to provide cross-sectional views

C. uses powerful magnet and radio waves to take images

D. uses high-frequency sound waves to view organs and structures in body

E. images developed based on energy emitted from radioactive substances

Case Studies

Case Study #1

Radiology Report

Left Ankle (two views): The left ankle shows no evidence of fracture or dislocation. The visualized bones and their respective articular surfaces are intact.

Conclusion: Normal left ankle

Index: X-ray, ankle 73600–73610

Code: 73600–LT Radiologic examination, ankle; two views

Case Study #2

X-ray of elbow, 3 views

Radiograph: Left elbow, 3 views

Indications: Pain in elbow after fall

Findings: There is a mildly displaced, slightly angulated fracture involving the supracondylar portion of the distal humerus. There is associated joint effusion reflecting hemarthrosis.

Index: X-ray, Elbow

Code: 73080–LT Radiological examination, elbow; complete, minimum of three views

Case Study #3

Bilateral Screening Mammogram

Comparison was made to multiple prior studies

Findings: Examination demonstrates moderately dense fibroglandular tissue. A nodular density is seen in the left central areolar region, which was seen on the prior studies and is essentially unchanged. There is no evidence of any suspicious calcifications. Skin and nipples have no abnormality. As compared with prior study, there is no significant interval change.

Impression: No radiographic evidence of malignancy. No significant interval change since prior study.

Index: Mammography, screening

Code: 77057 Screening mammography, bilateral

Case Study #4

CT Scan of the Head

Technique: Non-contrast CT scan of the head

Findings: No evidence of acute bleed is noted. The ventricles are not dilated and are maintained in their midline position. No evidence of any low attenuation area, especially in the basal ganglia or in the brainstem, noted to suggest acute or old infarct. The posterior fossa appears normal. No abnormal calcifications are seen.

Impression: No evidence of acute bleed identified. No midline shift or acute infarct noted.

Index: CT Scan, without contrast, Head

Code: 70450 Computed tomography, head or brain; without contrast material

Case Study #5

KUB, Upper GI Series

The KUB study reveals a large amount of fecal matter present in the colon. Staples are seen in the right upper quadrant. The stomach is high and transverse in type. There is a small sliding hiatal hernia and there is small gastroesophageal reflux. The duodenal bulb fills without ulceration. The stomach empties well.

Opinion: Small sliding hiatal hernia with intermittent gastrointestinal reflux.

Index: X-ray, Gastrointestinal Tract

Code: 74241 Radiological examination, gastrointestinal tract, upper; with or without delayed films, with KUB

Case Study #6

Upper Abdominal Ultrasound

The gall bladder, liver, pancreas, kidneys and spleen are well delineated and appear normal. The bile ducts are not distended. The abdominal aorta and inferior vena cava are normal in caliber.

Opinion: Normal upper abdominal sonogram

Index: Ultrasound, abdomen

Code: 76700 Ultrasound, abdominal, real time with image documentation; complete (See note before code that describes a complete examination.)

Case Study #7

Oral Cholecystogram

The gallbladder concentrates the contrast medium well and numerous radiolucent calculi are demonstrated.

Diagnosis: Cholelithiasis

> **Index: Cholecystography**
>
> **Code: 74290 Cholecystography, oral contrast**

Case Study #8

CT Scan, right elbow

Tomographic cuts were taken through the elbow at 3-mm intervals in AP and lateral views. No bone or joint abnormalities are evident. No fracture is evident.

Impression: Normal right elbow

> **Index: CT Scan, without Contrast, Arm**
>
> **Code: 73200–RT Computed tomography, upper extremity; without contrast**

Case Study #9

KUB and Intravenous Pyelogram

The KUB is normal. No urinary calcifications can be identified.

Following the intravenous injection, there is a good delineation of the urinary tract. The kidneys are small measuring 9.5 cm in their greatest length. The renal collecting system, ureters, and bladder appear normal.

Opinion: The kidneys measure slightly small. The urinary tract is otherwise normal.

> **Index: Pyelography**
>
> **Code: 74400 Urography (pyelography), intravenous, with or without KUB, with or without tomography**

Case Study #10

Chest X-ray

PA and lateral chest

The cardiopericardial silhouette and mediastinum are within normal limits. There is a left lower lobe infiltrate suspect for pneumonia. In addition, the right cardiac border is ill defined which may represent a right middle lobe infiltrate or atelectasis. There is surgical hardware of the lower cervical spine.

Impression: Left lower lobe infiltrate suspect for pneumonia. Probable right middle lobe infiltrate.

> **Index: X-ray, Chest (frontal view [referred to as posterior-anterior or PA], and the lateral [side] view.)**
>
> **Code: 71020 Radiologic examination, chest, two views, frontal and lateral**

Chapter 6
Pathology And Laboratory

Case Studies

Case Study #1

GENERAL CHEMISTRY

Sodium	Potassium	Chloride	Total CO$_2$	Glucose	BUN	Creatinine	Ionized Calcium
138	3.3	96	34	104	20	0.8	6.0

Index: Organ or Disease-Oriented Panel, Metabolic, Basic

Code: 80047 Basic Metabolic Panel

Case Study #2

Pathology Report

Specimen: Prostate Chips

Gross Examination: One specimen is received in formalin labeled with demographics and prostate chips. It consists of gray-tan, rubbery fragments of tissue measuring in aggregate 2.9 × 2.5 × 1.5 cm. The specimen is entirely submitted in cassettes A1-A4.

Microscopic Examination: Benign Prostatic Hypertrophy

Index: Pathology, Surgical, Gross and Micro Exam (scan range of codes 88302–88309)

Code: 88305 Level IV

Case Study #3

A stool sample is submitted to the lab for Helicobacter pylori

Index: Helicobacter Pylori, Stool

Code: 87338 Helicobacter pylori, stool

Case Study #4

A 55-year-old female is seen in the physician's office for an elevated blood pressure. She reports that there is a family history of kidney disease. A Cystatin C test is performed.

Index: Cystatin C, Blood

Code: 82610 Cystatin C

Case Study #5

A physician suspects that a patient might have an adrenocortical insufficiency and orders an insulin tolerance panel (Cortisol and Glucose) test.

Index: Insulin

Code: 80434 Insulin tolerance panel; for ACTH insufficiency

Case Study #6

Pathology Report

Specimen: Nasal Cyst

Gross Description: One specimen received in formalin labeled "nasal cyst." Skin measuring 1.7 × 0.8 × 0.5 cm. The specimen is serially sectioned revealing a 0.3 cm in diameter cyst containing white mucous-like material.

Microscopic Description: Skin, nose consistent with sebaceous adenoma

Index: Pathology, Surgical, Gross and Micro Exam (scan range of codes 88302–88309). Note that sebaceous adenoma is a benign cyst.

Code: 88304 Level III

Case Study #7

Lipid Panel

Test	Result	Reference Ranges
Cholesterol, serum	206	75–200
HDL	51	30–70
Triglycerides	119	20–250

Index: Organ or Disease-Oriented Panel, Lipid Panel

Code: 80061 Lipid Panel

Case Study #8

Urine Culture

Source: Straight Catheter

Abundant Gram Positive Cocci Suggestive of Streptococci

>100,000 CFU/ML Serratia Marcescens

>100,000 CFU/ML Enterococcus Species

Index: Culture, Bacteria, Urine

Code: 87086 Culture, bacterial; quantitative colony count, urine

Case Study #9

Test Name	Glycohemoglobin
Reference Range	3.6–6.8
Result	5.9

Index: Glycohemoglobin

Code: 83036 glycosylated (A1C)

Case Study #10

An 8-year-old girl presents in the urgent care center for abdominal pain associated with some diarrhea. The physician orders a fecal calprotectin test.

Index: Calprotectin, Fecal

Code: 83993 Calprotectin, fecal

Chapter 7
E/M

Case Study #1

The patient was seen in the physician's office after falling and injuring her ankle. The physician performed a brief HPI, a problem-focused exam and the decision-making was straightforward. What component(s) of the history is missing from this scenario?

ROS and PFSH

Case Study #2

A new patient is seen in the physician's office for dull ache in his left side. The physician performs a detailed history and physical examination and the medical decision-making was of moderate complexity. What is the correct E/M code for this service?

99203

Case Study #3

A 49-year-old established patient visits his family physician for a physical that is required by his place of employment. The physician documents a comprehensive history, exam and orders a series of routine tests, such as a chest X-ray and EKG. In addition, the physician counsels the patient about smoking habit. What CPT code would be selected to represent this service?

99396

Case Study #4

The physician documents that the patient has a cough, fever and muscle aches. A review of systems is performed, a detailed account of present illness is documented and the physician outlines the management options, complexity of treatment plan and orders tests. What key E/M component is missing from this documentation?

Physical exam

Case Study #5

A patient is seen on January 23, 2006 by a primary care physician who is a member of University Associates. A cardiologist (also a member of University Associates) sees the patient on November 24, 2007. Would the visit on November 24th be classified as a new or established patient?

New

Case Study #6

An established patient is seen in the physician's office for counseling after having an extremely high cholesterol reading and hypertension. Which range of codes would be used to select the appropriate CPT code for these services?

99212–99215

Case Study #7

The physician sees a patient in Sunny Acres Nursing Facility as a follow-up visit. The patient has a urinary tract infection that is not responding to medication. The physician documents a problem-focused interval history, expanded problem-focused exam and the medical decision-making was of moderate complexity. What is the correct CPT code assignment for this service?

99308

Case Study #8

A patient is seen in the Emergency Department for severe low back pain. The ED physician performs an expanded problem-focused history, problem-focused examination and the medical decision-making was of moderate complexity. What is the correct E/M code assignment for this service?

99281 (Need 3 out of 3 key components met or exceeded; the examination was only problem focused.)

Case Study #9

Physician documents that critical care services were provided to a 12-year-old patient for 90 minutes. What is the correct E/M code assignment for this service?

99291, 99292

Case Study #10

A 55-year-old patient (post Lasix surgery) visits a new ophthalmologist for extreme dry eyes. The physician performs an expanded problem-focused history and exam and prescribes eye drops as needed. What is the correct E/M code assignment for this service?

99202 (For a new patient, all 3 key components must be met.)

Chapter 8
Medicine

Case Studies

Case Study #1

A 35-year-old patient receives an IM injection of the Lyme disease vaccine.

> **Index:**
>> **Immunization Administration, One Vaccine/Toxoid**
>>
>> **Vaccines, Lyme Disease**
>
> **Codes:**
>> **90471 Immunization administration, IM, one vaccine**
>>
>> **90665 Lyme disease vaccine, adult dosage, for intramuscular use**

Case Study #2

A 45-year-old patient complains of sneezing, coughing and occasional episodes of wheezing. The physician wants to determine the cause of these allergic symptoms and performs 30 percutaneous skin tests.

> **Index: Allergy Tests, Skin Tests, Allergen Extract**
>
> **Code: 95004 Percutaneous tests**

Case Study #3

A 55-year-old patient with Type II diabetes mellitus e-mails her registered dietitian to ask advice about a adding a food product to her diet. The dietitian promptly responds to the question and keeps a record of this correspondence. The date of the last visit was two weeks ago.

> **Index: Online Internet Assessment and Management, Nonphysician**
>
> **Code: 98969 Online assessment and management service provided by qualified nonphysician health care professional to an established patient, guardian, or health care provider not originating from a related assessment and management service provided within the previous 7 days, using the Internet or similar electronic communications network.**

Case Study #4

A 45-year-old patient with end-stage renal disease (ESRD) is seen in the outpatient dialysis clinic for services on July 2, 5, 9, 15, 18, 21, 24, and 28.

> **Index: End-Stage Renal Disease Services**
>
> **Code: 90921 End-stage renal disease related services per full month; for patients twenty years of age and older**

Case Study #5

A 59-year-old female is undergoing chemotherapy treatment. She is seen in the clinic for a refill for her portable infusion pump.

Index: Infusion Pump, Maintenance

Code: 96521 Refilling and maintenance of portable pump

Case Study #6

A patient is seen in the Emergency Department with severe vomiting and diarrhea due to viral gastroenteritis. IV hydration is prescribed and takes one hour to administer.

Index: Hydration

Code: 90760 Intravenous infusion, hydration; initial, up to 1 hour

Case Study #7

Patient was diagnosed with actinic keratosis with lesions on several locations of the face. The patient receives irradiation of the areas with photodynamic therapy illuminator for 15 minutes.

Index: Photodynamic Therapy, External

Code: 96567 Photodynamic therapy

Case Study #8

A 67-year-old patient with multiple medical problems is currently taking six prescriptions and several over-the-counter agents. The primary care physician has a concern about side effects; therefore; the patient is referred to a pharmacist for assessment and management of medications. The pharmacist assesses the treatment and makes recommendations during the 10 minute face-to-face visit.

Index: Medication Therapy Management, Pharmacist Provided

Code: 99605 Medication therapy management service(s) provided by a pharmacist, individual, face-to-face with patient, with assessment and intervention if provided; initial 15 minutes, new patient

Case Study #9

A 32-year-old female is referred to the Behavioral Health Clinic due to significant personality changes. A series of tests is administered to evaluate the patient's emotionality, intellectual abilities, personality and psychopathology. The computerized test is completed in order to assist with establishing a diagnosis.

Index: Psychiatric Diagnosis, Psychological Testing, Computer-Assisted

Code: 96103 Psychological testing, administered by computer

Case Study #10

ELECTROENCEPTHALOGRAM

Complaint: Altered mental status

Current Medications: Vasotec, Lanoxin and Lasix

State of patient during recording: awake.

Description: The background is characterized by diffuse slowing and disorganization consisting of medium-voltage theta rhythm at 4–6 Hz seen from all head areas. From anterior head areas, faster activity at beta range. Eye movements and muscle artifacts are noted. Photic stimulation and hyperventilation were not performed. Total recording time was 40 minutes.

IMPRESSION: This is a moderately abnormal record due to diffuse slowing and disorganization of the background, with the slowing being at theta range.

Index: Electroencephalography

Code: 95816 EEG,; including recording awake and drowsy

Chapter 9
Anesthesia

Case Studies

Case Study #1

Patient admitted for uterine fibroids and dysmenorrhea. The surgeon performs a vaginal hysterectomy.

Index: Anesthesia, Hysterectomy, Vaginal

Code: 00944 Anesthesia, for vaginal procedures; vaginal hysterectomy

Case Study #2

Patient admitted for a right ureteral stent placement. Surgeon performs a cystoscopy with insertion of ureteral stent.

Index: Anesthesia, Urethrocystoscopy

Code: 00910 Anesthesia for transurethral procedures

Case Study #3

This is a 49-year-old man with a chronic right-sided submandibular swelling over the last few years. The diagnosis of right sialoadenitis was made. An excision of right submandibular gland was performed.

Index: Anesthesia, Salivary Gland

Code: 00100 Anesthesia for procedures on salivary glands, including biopsy

Case Study #4

Patient is being treated for a lateral meniscus tear. Surgeon performs an arthroscopy meniscectomy.

Index: Anesthesia, Arthroscopic Procedures, Knee

Code: 01382 Anesthesia for diagnostic arthroscopic procedures of knee joint

Case Study #5

The patient is a 65-year-old male who was recently treated for low anterior resection for a stage II superior rectal cancer. Adjuvant chemotherapy, planned. Placement of long-term venous access device was requested. Surgeon inserts a Port-a-Cath.

Index: Anesthesia, Central Venous Circulation

Code: 00532 Anesthesia for access to central venous circulation

Case Study #6

The patient is a 76-year-old male with substantial underlying pulmonary disease. He has required mechanical ventilation for approximately two to three weeks and failed several attempts to be completely taken off mechanical ventilation. He was brought to the operating room for placement of a tracheostomy tube.

Index: Anesthesia, trachea

Code: 00320 Anesthesia for all procedures on esophagus, thyroid, larynx, trachea and lymphatic system of neck; not otherwise specified, age 1 year or older

Case Study #7

The patient is a 56-year-old male who presented to the ENT Clinic with a history of left-sided nasal obstruction. The following procedures were performed: left maxillary sinusotomy, left anterior ethmoidectomy and removal of left nasal polyposis.

Index: Anesthesia, Nose

Code: 00160 Anesthesia for procedures on nose and accessory sinuses; not otherwise specified

Case Study #8

The patient is a 56-year-old man previously diagnosed with pancreatic cancer. The surgeon performs a partial excision of the pancreas.

Index: Anesthesia, Pancreatectomy

Code: 00794 Anesthesia for pancreatectomy, partial or total

Case Study #9

Patient has a diagnosis of urinary retention. The surgeon performs a transurethral resection of the prostate.

Index: Anesthesia, Transurethral Procedures

Code: 00914 Anesthesia for transurethral resection of prostate

Chapter 10
HCPCS

Case Studies

Identify the key term from the index and assign codes from the *HCPCS Level II* to the following cases.

Case Study #1

Clubfoot wedge to modify a shoe

> **Index: Clubfoot wedge**
>
> **Code: L3380 Clubfoot wedge**

Case Study #2

Patient with asthma requires a nebulizer with compressor

> **Index: Nebulizer**
>
> **Code: E0570 Nebulizer, with compressor**

Case Study #3

Patient has extreme dry eyes. Physician inserts temporary, absorbable lacrimal duct implants in each eye.

> **Index: Lacrimal duct implant, temporary**
>
> **Code: A4262 × 2 Temporary, absorbable lacrimal duct implant, each**

Case Study #4

Injection of 50 mg of progesterone

> **Index: Progesterone**
>
> **Code: J2675 Injection, progesterone, 50 mg**

Case Study #5

At-risk assessment for patient who is 10 weeks pregnant.

> **Index: Prenatal care**
>
> **Code: H1000 Prenatal care, at-risk assessment**

Case Study #6

Standard metal bed pan

Index: Bed, pan

Code: E0275 Bed pan, standard, metal or plastic

Case Study #7

Screening mammography, bilateral (direct digital image)

Index: Mammography

Code: G0202 Screening mammography, producing direct digital image, bilateral, all views

Case Study #8

Injection 500 mg vancomycin HC1

Index: Vancomycin

Code: J3370 Injection, vancomycin HC1, 500 mg

Case Study #9

IV pole for infusion

Index: IV Pole

Code: E0776 IV pole (note in the infusion supplies section)

Case Study #10

Arthroscopy of left knee for cartilage debridement of medial compartment and removal of loose bodies in lateral compartment.

Index: Arthroscopy, knee, removal of loose body

Code: G0289–LT Arthroscopy, knee, surgical, for removal of loose body, foreign body, debridement/shaving of articular cartilage at the time of other surgical knee arthroscopy in a different compartment of the same knee

Chapter 11
Reimbursement in the Ambulatory Setting

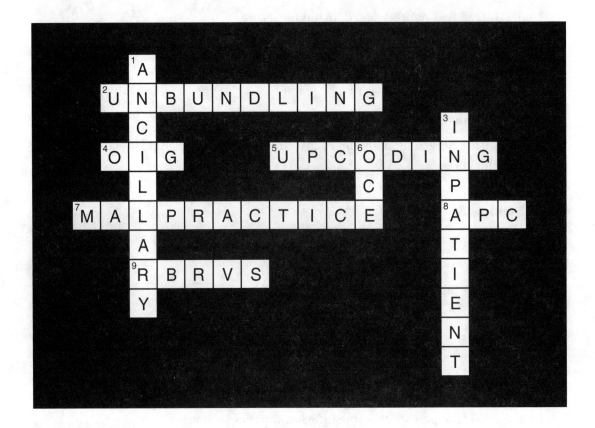

Across

2. Incorrectly assigning multiple codes [UNBUNDLING]

4. Develops yearly Workplan [OIG]

5. Assigning a code for higher payment [UPCODING]

7. RVU's include physician work, practice and _____ expenses [MALPRACTICE]

8. Reimbursement system for ambulatory surgery centers [APC]

9. Reimbursement system for physicians [RBRVS]

Down

1. Status indicator X identifies _____ services [ANCILLARY]

3. Status indicator C describes _____ procedures [INPATIENT]

6. Tool used to weed out incorrect claims [OCE]

Case Studies

Case Study #1—Medical Necessity

A 47-year-old female patient is seen in an outpatient setting for a variety of symptoms, including fatigue, weakness and insomnia. The physician orders the following tests:

```
FBS
PSA
WBC
T3, T4
TSH
```

Which test(s) does not meet medical necessity?

PSA (Prostate-Specific Antigen) would not be appropriate for a female patient.

Case Study #2—Use of Modifiers

1. _____ 28445 Open treatment of talus fracture, includes internal fixation, when performed

2. ✔ 28150 Phalangectomy, toe, each toe (**Need to append TA–T9 for toe specific HCPCS Level II Modifiers.**)

3. ✔ 11400 Excision, benign lesion including margins, except skin tag (unless listed elsewhere), trunk, arms, or legs; excised diameter 0.5 cm or less (**LT and RT modifiers are not appropriate on excision of lesion codes.**)

4. _____ 23500 Closed treatment of clavicular fracture; without manipulation

5. ✔ 71060 Bronchography, bilateral, radiological supervision and interpretation (**Description in CPT code states "bilateral"; therefore use of LT or RT is not appropriate.**)

Case Study #3—Medical Necessity

1. _____ R/O pregnancy (C)   A. spirometry

2. _____ low back pain (D)   B. EKG

3. _____ hearing loss (E)   C. Human chorionic gonadotropin (hCG)

4. _____ COPD (A)   D. osteopathic manipulative treatment

5. _____ coughing, sneezing, runny nose (F)   E. tympanometry

6. _____ tachycardia (B)   F. allergy tests